Chocolate to Morphine

Understanding Mind-Active Drugs

Andrew Weil, M.D.

and Winifred Rosen

Houghton Mifflin Company   Boston

Library of Congress Cataloging in Publication Data

Weil, Andrew.
  Chocolate to morphine.

  Includes index.
  1. Psychotropic drugs.   2. Drugs—Popular works.
I. Rosen, Winifred, date.   II. Title.
RM315.W44   1983   613.8   82-12112
ISBN 0-395-33108-0
ISBN 0-395-33190-0 pbk.

Printed in the United States of America

AL 10 9 8 7 6 5 4

Book design by Edith Allard, Designworks

Acknowledgments

Honey Williams and Budd Colby gave us the original idea for this book when they complained that they could not find anything good on the subject to give teen-agers to read.

Jeff Steingarten helped us in the early stages of our work, as did Woody Wickham and Norman Zinberg.

We are most fortunate to have had Anita McClellan as our editor at Houghton Mifflin. Her energetic support and suggestions have been invaluable.

We are much indebted to Dr. Michael Aldrich and the Fitz Hugh Ludlow Memorial Library in San Francisco for assistance in finding illustrations for the text. Jeremy Bigwood also provided illustrations, as well as good suggestions and needed infusions of energy. Special thanks go to Zig Schmitt for his company, support, and help in finding published source materials.

Leif Zerkin, editor of the *Journal of Psychoactive Drugs*, came up with recommendations for additional reading and some good cartoons. Ken and Maria Robbins provided photographs, food, and information. Dody Fugate of the University of Arizona gave us outstanding photographic service.

Friends who helped us complete the manuscript include Richard Carey, Howard Kotler, Dr. David Smith, Sara Davidson, Helen Shewman, Dr. Tod Mikuriya, Jake Myers, Jonathan Meader, Sue Fleishman, Tim Plowman, and Stanley and Jenine Moss.

We thank Dr. Richard Evans Schultes and the staff of the Harvard Botanical Museum for their help with illustrations and Karen Frankian and Signe Warner at Houghton Mifflin for their part in tying together the many pieces of this work.

Many drugs mentioned in this book have three names: a chemical name that describes the molecule, a generic or common name, and a brand name owned by a company that markets the drug. For example, Valium is the brand name of a tranquilizer whose generic name is diazepam. The chemical name of this same drug is 7-chloro-1,3-dihydro-1-methyl-5-phenyl-2H-1,4-benzodiazepin-2-one.

Because chemical names are long and cumbersome and useful only to chemists, we do not give them. We have tried to stick to generic names, which are printed in lower-case letters and followed, when relevant, by the most common brand names, enclosed in parentheses and capitalized. Thus: diazepam (Valium).

If the brand name is much better known than the generic name, as in the case of Valium, we will use it to refer to the drug after the first reference. Many "street" drugs, such as cocaine, LSD, and marijuana, do not have brand names.

We have selected comments about mind-active drugs and accounts of experiences with them from users and nonusers of all ages. Short excerpts from many of these selections appear in the margins of the text. For fuller transcripts, see the appendix, beginning on page 181.

Contents

Chocolate to Morphine

Straight Talk at the Start

DRUGS ARE HERE TO STAY.
History teaches that it is vain to hope that drugs will ever disappear and that any effort to eliminate them from society is doomed to failure.

During most of this century, Western society has attempted to deal with its drug problems through negative actions: by various wars on drug abuse implemented by repressive laws, outrageous propaganda, and attacks on users, suppliers, and sources of disapproved substances. These wars have been consistently lost. More people are taking more drugs now than ever before. Drug use has invaded all classes and ethnic groups and has spread to younger and younger children. Also, more people *abuse* drugs now than ever before, and the drug laws have directly created ugly and ever-enlarging criminal networks that corrupt society and cause far worse damage than the substances they distribute.

The authors of this book were teen-agers and college students in the 1960s. They had to confront the explosion of drug use of that era and find out for themselves the benefits and dangers of substances they never learned about at home or in school. One of us — Andrew Weil — has since become a professional researcher of drugs. He has a medical degree from Harvard and a rich background of travel among drug-using cultures in other parts of the world, from the deserts of east Africa to the jungles of South America. He draws on his training and his professional and personal experience with most of the substances described in these pages. As a recognized expert, he is frequently invited to lecture on drugs to audiences of doctors as well as students, to testify on drugs in court trials, to write about them for textbooks and popular magazines, and to consult about them with government officials.

The other of us — Winifred Rosen — is a writer. She is the author of more than a dozen books for young people. The daughter of a psychoanalyst, she has long been interested in psychology and mental health. A former high-school teacher and a veteran of the 1960s who is open and articulate about her own experiences, she has talked extensively about drugs with people both old and young and can answer the questions of users and nonusers alike.

We have been writing and traveling together on and off ever since we first met in San Francisco in 1968 (where we both served for a time as volunteers in the Haight-Ashbury Free Medical Clinic). Both of us believe that the present drug problem can only change for the better if society alters its strategy drastically. In this book we are not going to argue for or against drugs and will not side with either those who endorse them or those who oppose them. Instead, we will follow a middle course by presenting neutral information and by asking both sides to change some basic conceptions about drugs as a result of reading this material.

At the outset, we will insist that readers learn to distinguish drug use from drug abuse. As long as society continues to call all those who take disapproved substances "drug abusers," it will have an insoluble problem of enormous proportions. Real drug abusers are those in bad relationships with drugs,* whether the drugs are approved or disapproved by society, and unfortunately little can be done to help them. Once people get into bad relationships with drugs it is very hard to get them out. For most abusers the only practical choice is total abstinence or continued abuse. (Some people may prefer to see heroin addicts in methadone treatment rather than seeking heroin on the street, but let us not kid ourselves: the "treatment" is just addiction to another narcotic.)

If society cannot do much about drug abuse once it develops, it certainly can, and should, work to *prevent* abuse. Instead of wasting so much time, money, and energy fighting the hopeless battle against existing drug abuse, society must begin to help people avoid becoming abusers in the first place.

*See Chapter 4.

Preventing drug abuse *is* a realistic goal. Two approaches are possible. One is to teach people, especially young people, how to satisfy their needs and desires without recourse to drugs. The second is to teach people how to form good relationships with drugs so that if they choose to use drugs, they will continue to be users and never become abusers.

The burden of this task will fall mainly upon parents and secondarily upon teachers; it is not a process that can be mandated by law or accomplished by public policy. However, laws and public policies must not undermine the work of parents and teachers by perpetuating irrational ideas about drugs, ideas rooted in fear and prejudice.* The kind of instruction we would like to see will bear no resemblance to what is called "drug education" today. Drug education as it now exists is, at best, a thinly disguised attempt to scare young people away from disapproved drugs by greatly exaggerating the dangers of these substances. More often than not, lectures, pamphlets, and film strips that take this approach stimulate curiosity, make the prohibited substances look more attractive to the audience, and make authorities appear ridiculous.

Parents and teachers will probably be comfortable with efforts to interest children in alternatives to drugs. It will be harder to support programs that teach young people how to form good relationships with drugs. Nevertheless, with drugs so available and with children so disposed to experiment with them, this kind of teaching is vital. Young people are going to decide for themselves whether to use drugs. The most that responsible adults can hope to do is give children the information that will enable them to use drugs intelligently if they choose to use them at all.

We have tried to make this book accessible to young people by keeping our language and ideas simple and straightforward. When we were growing up, information like this was not available to the general public. As teen-agers, we struggled to get the facts, making many mistakes in the difficult process of learning the effects of drugs and adopting rules for living with them. We know how hard it is to grow up in a drug-filled world and hope our experience will be of use to younger generations.

To our teen-age readers we offer some general advice at the start:

You are growing up in a world well stocked with drugs. All of them can be used wisely or stupidly. Grownups will give you

*See Chapter 2.

much misinformation about them and will often be dishonest or hypocritical about their own drug use.* You will see many of your acquaintances become involved with drugs and will have many opportunities to experiment with them yourself if you have not already done so. The fact that grownups lie to you about the dangers of drugs they disapprove of does not mean those drugs have no dangers. *All drugs are dangerous.*

The only way you can be absolutely sure of avoiding problems with drugs is never to use them. That is a perfectly reasonable choice and may allow you more freedom than your drug-taking peers. Keep it in mind if you find yourself under pressure to take drugs. You may feel left out of certain groups if you abstain, but you will not really be missing anything. All of the experiences people have with drugs can be had in other ways.† If you do decide to experiment with drugs, whether approved or disapproved, make sure you know what the drugs are, where they come from, how they are likely to affect your body, and what precautions you should take to contain their potential for harm.** Remember that forming good relationships with drugs requires awareness and practice. Don't use drugs unconsciously and don't spend time around people who do.

If you involve yourself with illegal drugs, keep in mind the terrible consequences that being arrested can bring to you and your family. On the other hand, do not make the mistake of supposing that just because a drug is legal it is safe. Some of the strongest and most dangerous drugs are legal.

You are less likely to encounter problems if you take dilute forms of natural drugs by mouth on occasion, especially if you take them for positive reasons according to rules you set for yourself.‡ You are more likely to get into trouble if you take concentrated drugs frequently, particularly if you take them to escape feelings of unhappiness or boredom, or just because the drugs happen to be around.

It is a bad idea to take drugs in school. Even if school bores you, you have to be there, and mastering classroom skills is your ticket to freedom and independence in adult life. Drugs can interfere with your education by making it hard to pay attention, concentrate, and remember, or by involving you with people who reinforce negative attitudes about school.

*See Chapter 2.

†See Chapter 13.

**See Chapters 6–11.

‡See Chapter 4.

Drugs are likely to be a source of friction between you and your parents. If your parents get upset with you for taking drugs, consider that they might have good reasons, such as valid fears about your safety, health, or psychological growth. Be willing to talk honestly with them and to hear their side with an open mind. Think about how you would feel in their place. What advice would you give your child if you found out he was taking drugs? Question your parents about the drugs they use. Maybe they will agree to give up theirs if you will give up yours. Try to see what your experiences have in common with theirs. What alternatives to drug use can your parents suggest? If you can convince them that your drug use is responsible, you may be able to allay their anxiety. If their fears come from ignorance or misinformation, try to educate them, not by being emotional but by being well informed about the drugs you use. Give them this book to read as a background to your discussions of drug use.

Finally, remember that wanting to feel high is not a symptom of mental illness or an unhealthy need to escape from reality. It is normal to want to vary your consciousness.* Drugs are just one way of doing it, though, and if you come to rely on them before you are grown up, you may not be able to appreciate a whole range of nondrug experiences that are more subtle but more rewarding over time. There is no question that drugs can get you high, but they are difficult to master and may fail you if you take them regularly.†

We hope that parents will read this book and use the information in it to help their children. We sympathize with parents today. You are much more likely than your own parents to have to confront the issue of a child's involvement with drugs. Before you react to the discovery that a son or daughter is using drugs, you should keep several points in mind:

A period of experimentation with drugs is today a normal phase of adolescence — a rite of passage that most children pass through unscathed.

Be sure you have accurate information about the drugs your child is using before you attempt to give advice. Children now are often well informed and contemptuous of antidrug information they know to be false. Insisting that marijuana leads to

*See Chapter 3.

†See Chapter 13.

heroin* or that LSD breaks chromosomes† is a sure way to lose a child's attention and respect for your credibility about drug use.

Examine your own drug use before you question your child's. If your relationships with alcohol, tobacco, caffeine, and tranquilizers are not as good as they might be, a position against drug use may have little impact on your child. If you use illegal substances, your stand is further weakened by your own violation of drug laws.

It is important to create a climate of trust in which you and your child can communicate openly about difficult subjects like sex and drugs. Good communication is impossible when a parent assumes the role of detective, police officer, judge, or warden.

As we will stress throughout this book, a drug user is not necessarily a drug abuser. Meet your drug-using child with an open mind. Try to remember how you felt as a teen-ager. What forbidden activities did you engage in, and how easy was it for you to discuss them with your parents when you were discovered? Remember that though the specific issues change from generation to generation, the basic conflicts and problems between adolescents and parents are universal and remarkably constant.

The primary responsibility for preventing drug abuse in your child is yours. Providing models of intelligent drug use is the best way to assure that your child will use drugs rather than abuse them (if he uses them at all). It is well known that alcoholics tend to come from families where one or both parents are alcoholic, but it is less well known that alcoholics also tend to come from families where both parents are teetotalers. Apparently the absence of a parental role model for successful drinking is the determining factor. The low incidence of alcoholism among Jews has long been ascribed to the integration of occasional social and ritual use of alcohol into Jewish family life.

We have seen parents in good relationships with marijuana let their children take occasional puffs of joints in much the same way that some Jewish parents allow their children ceremonial sips of wine. By not making these substances forbidden and therefore attractive, such parents reduce the chance that their children will use them in rebellious and destructive ways. This is not to say that you should introduce your child to every

*See page 120.

†See page 97.

drug mentioned in this book, or to any drug at all. Rather, the more you encourage openness within your home about drug use and the better your own relationships are with the drugs you use, the more effective you will be at passing healthy drug attitudes and habits on to your child.

Make rules and set limits for your child about drugs. If your child respects you and the ways you use alcohol, caffeine, and other substances, he or she will welcome guidelines. Be realistic about the rules you make. For example, if you feel strongly that you do not want illegal drugs in the house, you should certainly insist that your child not bring them home. Of course, you must realize that your son or daughter may then use illegal substances outside the house. The choice is yours.

Keep in mind that the main reason children experiment with drugs is to experience other states of consciousness.* High states appeal to young people as much as they do to adults. Grownups enjoy racing cars and boats, hang-gliding, dancing, drinking, smoking, and many other consciousness-changing activities. Don't make your child feel it is wrong to get high. If you oppose the use of drugs to do it, be prepared to forgo your own drug use as an example to your child. Consistency and honesty are crucial if parents are to gain real credibility with children. Also, be prepared to suggest alternatives if you are opposed to drugs.† Alcohol is not an alternative. It, too, is a drug, and the advantage of its legality is more than offset by its many dangers for users of any age.**

Finally, consider the parallel problem of sexual experimentation, which, like drugs, is an adolescent rite of passage parents have to deal with. Is it better to provide support for your child by expressing trust and offering reliable information about these issues or to force your child to seek information and experience without guidance and in risky ways? We believe the first course to be the better one, in matters concerning sex and drugs alike.

Both of us have taught in schools and colleges and are aware that schools are now popular places for the distribution and consumption of drugs. We know that teachers are likely to be distressed by the prevalence of drug use among children today, especially when they encounter increasing numbers of students

*See Chapter 3.

†See Chapter 13.

**See pages 60–68.

who cannot concentrate and have trouble learning because they are intoxicated on one substance or another.

Teachers have a special role in influencing children, but when they have to talk about heated, emotional subjects like drugs, they must bow to so many pressures that often they cannot follow intuition or conscience. Teachers must frequently present drug education programs based on incorrect information and irrational attitudes. Acknowledging the falsity of the information may gain them the respect of students and allow them to influence drug use for the better, but it may also cost the teachers their jobs. We would like to see teachers inform themselves about drugs and work within the limits imposed on them to make classrooms places where young people feel free to discuss interest in, experiences with, and conflicts about drugs.

Just as with successful sex education, to do so teachers will have to clarify their own attitudes and be prepared to answer questions about their own uses and habits, since students will certainly ask. As in parental discussions of sex and drugs with teen-agers, honesty and consistency are required for teachers to have credibility with their students. Given the political dimensions of the drug controversy, many teachers may just want to avoid the whole issue. We cannot blame them, since we know how vulnerable their positions are. Still, because teachers can contribute so much toward the prevention of drug abuse, we hope they will try to find ways to change attitudes for the better.

Although we have written this book so that young people can read it, we intend it for doctors, lawmakers, members of the clergy, teachers, and users and nonusers regardless of age. We have gathered this information from many sources, including our own experience, and, whenever possible, we have included first-person observations by others to create a more balanced overall picture. We have tried throughout to indicate how society can work to prevent drug abuse by encouraging the use of alternatives to drugs and encouraging the formation of good relationships with drugs when people choose to use them.

2

What Is a Drug?

MOST PEOPLE WOULD AGREE that heroin is a drug. It is a white powder that produces striking changes in the body and mind in tiny doses. But is sugar a drug? Sugar is also a white powder that strongly affects the body, and some experts say it affects mental function and mood as well. Like heroin, it can be addicting. How about chocolate? Most people think of it as a food or flavor, but it contains a chemical related to caffeine, is a stimulant, and can also be addicting. Is salt a drug? Many people think they cannot live without it, and it has dramatic effects on the body.

A common definition of the word *drug* is any substance that in small amounts produces significant changes in the body, mind, or both. This definition does not clearly distinguish drugs from some foods. The difference between a drug and a poison is also unclear. All drugs become poisons in high enough doses, and many poisons are useful drugs in low enough doses. Is alcohol a food, a drug, or a poison? The body can burn it as a fuel, just like sugar or starch, but it causes intoxication and can kill in overdose. Many people who drink alcohol crusade against drug abuse, never acknowledging that they themselves are involved with a powerful drug. In the same way, many cigarette addicts have no idea that tobacco is a very strong drug, and few people who drink coffee realize the true nature of that beverage.

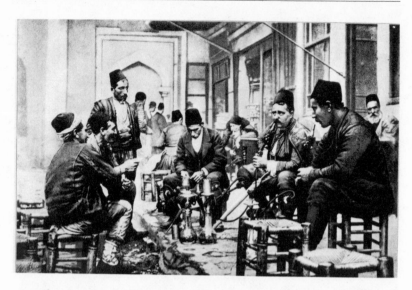

Turkish men smoking tobacco in water pipes in a Constantinople coffee house, about 1900. (Courtesy of the Swiss Federal Institute of Technology)

The decision to call some substances drugs and others not is often arbitrary. In the case of medical drugs — substances such as penicillin, used only to treat physical illness — the distinction may be easier to make. But talking about psychoactive drugs — substances that affect mood, perception, and thought — is tricky.

In the first place, foods, drugs, and poisons are not clear-cut categories. Second, people have strong emotional reactions to them. Food is good. Poison is bad. Drugs may be good or bad, and whether they are seen as good or bad depends on who is looking at them. Many people agree that drugs are good when doctors give them to patients in order to make them better. Some religious groups, such as Christian Scientists, do not share that view, however. They believe that God intends us to deal with illness without drugs.

When people take psychoactive drugs on their own, in order to change their mood or feel pleasure, the question of good or bad gets even thornier. The whole subject of pleasure triggers intense controversy. Should pleasure come as a reward for work or suffering? Should people feel guilty if they experience pleasure without suffering for it in some way? Should work itself be unpleasant? These questions are very important to us, but they do not have easy answers. Different people and different cultures answer them in different ways.

Drug use is universal. Every human culture in every age of history has used one or more psychoactive drugs. (The one exception is the Eskimos, who were unable to grow drug plants

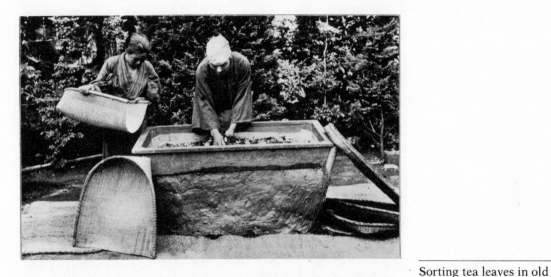

Sorting tea leaves in old Japan. (Courtesy of the Swiss Federal Institute of Technology)

and had to wait for white men to bring them alcohol.) In fact, drug-taking is so common that it seems to be a basic human activity. Societies must come to terms with people's fascination with drugs. Usually the use of certain drugs is approved and integrated into the life of a tribe, community, or nation, sometimes in formal rituals and ceremonies. The approval of some drugs for some purposes usually goes hand in hand with the disapproval of other drugs for other purposes. For example, some early Muslim sects encouraged the use of coffee in religious rites, but had strict prohibitions against alcohol. On the other hand, when coffee came to Europe in the seventeenth century, the Roman Catholic Church opposed it as an evil drug but continued to regard wine as a traditional sacrament.

Everybody is willing to call certain drugs bad, but there is little agreement from one culture to the next as to which these are. In our own society, all nonmedical drugs other than alcohol, tobacco, and caffeine are viewed with suspicion by the majority. There are subgroups within our society, however, that hold very different opinions. Many North American Indians who use peyote and tobacco in religious rituals consider alcohol a curse. The most fervent members of the counterculture that arose in the 1960s regard marijuana and psychedelics as beneficial while rejecting not only alcohol, tobacco, and coffee but most other legal and illegal drugs as well. Classic heroin addicts, or junkies, may reject psychedelics and marijuana as dangerous but think of narcotics as desirable and necessary. Some yogis in India use marijuana ritually, but teach that opiates and alcohol are harmful. Muslims may tolerate the use of opium, marijuana, and qat (a strongly stimulating leaf), but are very strict in their exclusion of alcohol.

Furthermore, attitudes about which drugs are good or bad tend to change over time within a given culture. When tobacco first came to Europe from the New World it provoked such strong opposition that authorities in some countries tried to stamp it out by imposing the death penalty for users. But within a century its use was accepted and even encouraged in the belief that it made people work more efficiently. In this century Americans' attitudes toward alcohol have shifted from nonchalant tolerance to antagonism strong enough to result in national prohibition, and back to near-universal acceptance. The current bitter debate over marijuana is mostly a conflict between an older generation that views the drug as evil and a younger generation that finds it preferable to alcohol.

Students of behavior tell us that dividing the world into good and evil is a fundamental human need. The existence of evil provokes fear and demands explanation. Why is there sickness? Why is there death? Why do crops fail? Why is there war? And, most important, how should we act to contain evil and avoid disaster? One attempt at a solution is to attribute evil to external things, and then prohibit, avoid, or try to destroy them. This is how taboos arise.

People tend to create taboos about the activities and substances that are most important to them. Food, sex, and pleasure are very important, and many taboos surround them — although, again, there is little agreement from culture to culture as to what is good and what is bad. Muslims and Jews eat beef but not pork; some groups in India eat pork but not beef. Homosexuality is taboo in most modern Western cultures, but has been fully accepted in the past and is still accepted today in certain parts of the world.

People who adhere to taboos justify them with logical reasons. Jews like to think they do not eat pork because pigs are unclean and may have carried disease in former times. Christians argue that homosexuality is a sin because it perverts God's intended use of sex for procreation. Actually, reasons for taboos are secondary; the basic process is the dividing of important things into good and evil — a form of magical thinking that tries to gain control over sources of fear. The reasons and justifications come later.

Because psychoactive drugs can give pleasure and can change the ways people think, perceive the world, behave, and relate to each other, they invite magical thinking and taboos. When you hear arguments on the merits or dangers of drugs, even by scientific experts, remember that these may be secondary justifications of pre-existing views that are deep-seated and rooted in emotion. (It is always easy for both sides to produce statistics and "scientific evidence" to support opposing views.)

Because drugs are so connected with people's fears and desires, it is very hard to find neutral information on them. In this book we try to give unbiased facts about all psychoactive drugs people are likely to encounter today. We cannot say that we have no biases about drugs, but we think we know what they are. Our strongest conviction is that drugs themselves are neither good nor bad; rather, they are powerful substances that can be put to good or bad uses. We are concerned with the relationships people form with drugs, whether legal or illegal, approved or unapproved. We believe that by presenting neutral information about these substances, we can help people, especially young people, come to terms with drugs. Our purpose is not to encourage or discourage the use of any drug, but rather to help people learn to live in a world where drugs exist and not get hurt by them.

Suggested Reading

The best book on the subject of how societies classify drugs as good and evil is *Ceremonial Chemistry: The Ritual Persecution of Drugs, Addicts, and Pushers* by Thomas Szasz (Garden City, New York: Doubleday/Anchor, 1975). Szasz is a psychiatrist interested in the assumptions that lead people to call some kinds of behavior sick or wrong. His discussion of drugs and drug users as scapegoats is excellent.

A book written for junior-high and high-school students that gives a good overview of the subject is *Mind Drugs* (third edition) edited by Margaret O. Hyde (New York: McGraw-Hill, 1974).

3

Why People Use Drugs

DRUGS ARE FASCINATING because they can change our awareness. The basic reason people take drugs is to vary their conscious experience. Of course there are many other ways to alter consciousness, such as listening to music, making music, dancing, fasting, chanting, exercising, surfing, meditating, falling in love, hiking in the wilderness (if you live in a city), visiting a city (if you live in the wilderness), having sex, daydreaming, watching fireworks, going to a movie or play, jumping into cold water after taking a hot sauna, participating in religious rituals. The list is probably endless, and includes nearly all the activities that people put most of their time, energy, and hard-earned money into. This suggests that changing consciousness is something people like to do.

Human beings, it seems, are born with a need for periodic variations in consciousness. The behavior of young children supports this idea. Infants rock themselves into blissful states; many children discover that whirling, or spinning, is a powerful technique to change awareness; some also experiment with hyperventilation (rapid, deep breathing) followed by mutual chest-squeezing or choking, and tickling to produce paralyzing laughter. Even though these practices may produce some un-

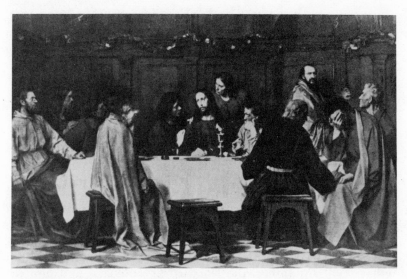

comfortable results, such as dizziness or nausea, the whole experience is so reinforcing that children do it again and again, often despite parental objections. Since children all over the world engage in these activities, the desire to change consciousness does not seem to be a product of a particular culture but rather to arise from something basically human. As children grow older they find that certain available substances put them in similar states. The attractiveness of drugs is that they provide an easy, quick route to these experiences.

Wine is used ceremonially in both Judaic and Christian rites. According to the Gospels, the Last Supper was the Jewish Passover feast. (Free Lance Photographers Guild)

Many drug users talk about getting high. Highs are states of consciousness marked by feelings of euphoria, lightness, self-transcendence, concentration, and energy. People who never take drugs also seek out highs. In fact, having high experiences from time to time may be necessary to our physical and mental health, just as dreaming at night seems to be vital to our well-being. Perhaps that is why a desire to alter normal consciousness exists in everyone and why people pursue the experiences even though there are sometimes uncomfortable side effects.

Although the desire for high states is at the root of drug-taking in both children and grownups, people also take drugs for other, more practical reasons. These include:

To aid religious practices. Throughout history, people have used drug-induced states to transcend their sense of separateness and feel more at one with nature, God, and the supernatural. Marijuana was used for this purpose in ancient India, and many psychedelic plants are still so used today by Indians

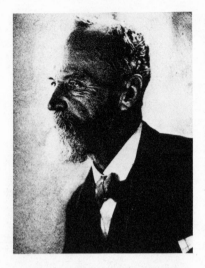

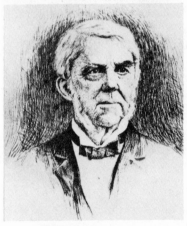

Top: William James (1842–1910), American psychologist and philosopher. (From *The Letters of William James*, edited by Henry James. Boston: Atlantic Monthly Press, 1920)

Bottom: Oliver Wendell Holmes (1809–1894), American writer and physician. (From *Medicine: An Historical Outline*, copyright 1931 by the Williams & Wilkins Co., Baltimore)

in North and South America. Alcohol has been used for religious purposes in many parts of the world; the role of wine in Roman Catholic and Judaic rites persists as an example. Among primitive people, psychoactive plants are often considered sacred — gifts from gods and spirits to unite people with the higher realms.

To explore the self. Curious individuals throughout history have taken psychoactive substances to explore and investigate parts of their own minds not ordinarily accessible. One of the most famous modern examples was the British writer and philosopher Aldous Huxley, who experimented extensively with mescaline in the 1950s. He left us a record of his investigations in a book called *The Doors of Perception.* Some other well-known "explorers" are Oliver Wendell Holmes, the nineteenth-century American physician, poet, and author, who experimented with ether; William James, the Harvard psychologist and philosopher of the late nineteenth century, who used nitrous oxide; Sigmund Freud, the father of psychoanalysis, who took cocaine; William S. Burroughs, a contemporary American novelist and user of opiates; Richard Alpert (Ram Dass), a psychologist and guru, who has extensive experience with LSD and other psychedelics; and John Lilly, a medical researcher and philosopher, who has experimented with ketamine. Many others who have followed this path have done so privately, keeping their experiences to themselves, or sharing them only with intimate companions.

To alter moods. Many people take drugs to relieve anxiety, depression, lethargy, or insomnia, or to escape from pain and boredom. The idea that unwanted moods are disease states treatable by taking medicines has become very popular in our society. The pharmaceutical industry has both encouraged and capitalized on this notion, with the result that the majority of legal medical drugs sold today are aimed at changing undesired moods. Young people see their parents use drugs in this way and are also influenced by advertising that directly promotes such behavior. Many people of all ages use nonmedical drugs, both legal and illegal ones, in this fashion.

To treat disease. Because psychoactive drugs really make people feel different, doctors and patients have always relied heavily on them for dealing with the symptoms of illness. Opium, morphine, and alcohol were mainstays of nineteenth-century medicine, used to treat everything from menstrual cramps to epilepsy. (One eminent physician of the day even called morphine "God's own medicine.") Tincture of marijuana was also a popular remedy. At the end of the nineteenth century, cocaine was promoted as a miracle drug and cure-all, and coca wine was the most widely prescribed drug for a time. In recent years, diazepam (Valium) has held that distinction. This kind of treatment may work by distracting a patient's attention from symptoms and shifting it instead toward the good feeling of a high. Sometimes the medical problem will then go away on its own. Often, however, if there is no treatment of the underlying cause of the symptoms, the problem will persist and the patient may go on to use the drug again and again until dependence results.

To promote and enhance social interaction.   "Let's have a drink" is one of the most frequent phrases in use today. It is an invitation to share time and communication around the consumption of a psychoactive drug. Like sharing food, taking drugs together is a ritual excuse for intimacy; coffee breaks and cocktail ("happy") hours are examples of the way approved drugs are used for this purpose. Disapproved drugs may draw people together even more strongly by establishing a bond of common defiance of authority. At the big rock concerts and Vietnam War protests of the 1960s, strangers often became instant comrades simply by passing a joint back and forth.

In different cultures other drugs perform the same function. For example, South American Indians take coca breaks together, much as we take coffee breaks, and chewing coca leaves with a friend establishes an important social bond. For South Sea Islanders, drinking kava in groups at night is the equivalent of an American cocktail party.

Aside from the ritual significance with which drugs are invested, their pharmacological effects may also enhance social interaction. Because alcohol lowers inhibitions in most people, businessmen and women have drinks at lunch to encourage openness and congeniality. Similarly, on dates people often drink to reduce anxiety and feelings of awkwardness. By producing alertness and euphoria, stimulants, such as cocaine, promote easy conversation, even among strangers.

So important is this function of psychoactive drugs that many people would find it difficult to relate to others if deprived of them.

To enhance sensory experience and pleasure.   Human beings are pleasure-seeking animals who are very inventive when it comes

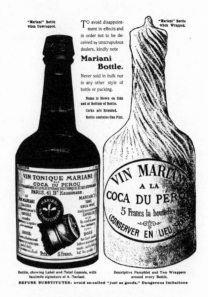

Mariani wine, containing an extract of Peruvian coca leaves, was made in Paris in the late 1800s and became the most popular medical prescription in the world, used by kings, queens, leaders of society, and at least one pope. (From the Vin Mariani Album of 1901, Beneficial Plant Research Association Reprint Edition, 1981; courtesy of Fitz Hugh Ludlow Memorial Library)

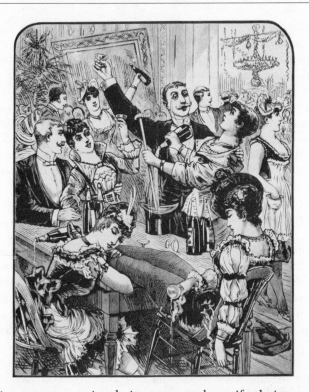

(Fitz Hugh Ludlow Memorial Library)

to finding ways to excite their senses and gratify their appetites. One of the characteristics of sensory pleasure is that it becomes dulled with repetition, and there are only so many ways of achieving pleasure. As much time, thought, and energy have gone into sex as into any human activity, but the possibilities of sexual positions and techniques are limited. By making people feel different, psychoactive drugs can make familiar experiences new and interesting again. The use of drugs in combination with sex is as old as the hills, as is drug use with such activities as dancing, eating, and listening to or playing music. Drinking wine with meals is an example of this behavior that dates back to prehistory and is still encouraged by society. Some men say that a good cigar and a glass of brandy make a fine meal complete. Pot lovers say that turning on is the perfect way for a fine meal to begin. Psychedelic drugs, especially, are intensifiers of experience and can make a sunset more fascinating than a movie. (Of course, psychedelics can also turn an unpleasant situation into a living nightmare.) Because drugs can, temporarily at least, make the ordinary extraordinary, many people seek them out and consume them in an effort to get more enjoyment out of life.

To stimulate artistic creativity and performance.   Writers have traditionally used psychoactive substances as sources of inspiration. The English poet Coleridge's famous visionary poem "Kubla Khan" was a transcription of one of his opium dreams. The French poet Charles Baudelaire took hashish as well as opium for creative inspiration. His compatriot, the novelist Alexandre Dumas, joined him in experiments with hashish. The American writer Edgar Allan Poe relied on opiates; some of the weirdness of his tales probably derives from his drug experiences. Sigmund Freud's early writings were inspired by cocaine; for a time he actively promoted cocaine as a miracle drug. Innumerable novelists, poets, playwrights, and journalists have found their inspiration in alcohol. Many have paid the high price of becoming alcoholics.

Some traditional peoples turn psychedelic visions into art. For example, the yarn paintings of the Huichol Indians of Mexico come directly from peyote sessions. Other artists find visions in their own imagination but use psychoactive drugs to help

In Xanadu did Kubla Khan
A stately pleasure dome decree:
Where Alph, the sacred river,
*   ran*
Through caverns measureless
*   to man*
Down to a sunless sea.
— opening lines of "Kubla Khan" (1798), by Samuel Taylor Coleridge (1772–1834)

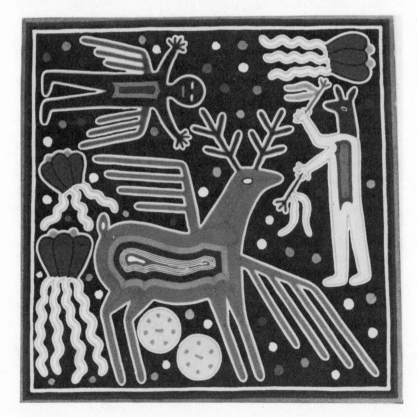

A Huichol yarn painting, showing the sacred deer, spirits, and three peyote plants. (Dody Fugate)

them do the work of translating their visions into art. Diego Rivera, the best-known Mexican artist of the twentieth century, was a user of marijuana. The famous American abstract painter Jackson Pollock was an alcoholic; he died at age forty-four in a car crash, the result of driving while intoxicated.

When marijuana first surfaced in America in the 1920s, musicians were among its most enthusiastic users, and many still use it today, both to compose and to perform. Some of the best-known jazz musicians have been heroin addicts.

There has been little scientific study of the relationship between drugs and creativity. Possibly, high states permit some people to view the world in novel perspectives and to gain insights they can later express artistically.

To improve physical performance.   Various drugs enable some people to perform out-of-the-ordinary feats. In the ancient Inca empire of Peru, relay runners used coca in order to be able to cover vast distances in the high Andes, carrying news and messages to all parts of the kingdom. Warriors throughout history have fortified themselves with alcohol before battle to boost their courage and decrease sensitivity to pain. Many professional athletes today follow in this tradition: baseball players chew tobacco; football and basketball players often take amphetamines and cocaine. Also, truckers will often complete long drives on little sleep and a lot of amphetamines.

To rebel.   Because drugs are so surrounded by taboos, they invite rebellious behavior. Breaking taboos is an obvious way to challenge the values of the "establishment." Children quickly learn they can upset parents, teachers, doctors, and other grown-up authorities by taking forbidden substances. Adolescence usually entails the assertion of independence, often by rejecting parental values. It is not surprising that adolescence is also a time of frequent experimentation with drugs. Unfortunately, our society's attempt to control drug-taking by making some substances illegal plays into the hands of rebellious children. Even some older people who have not entirely outgrown adolescent traits express rebelliousness in the ways they take drugs.

To go along with peer pressure.   Many people who would not seek out drugs on their own take them to go along with the crowd. A man or woman who does not drink with business colleagues is likely to feel like a freak. Some teen-agers start

---

You get into heroin because you have a lot of money in your pocket, and you can't go to video games all the time, and you think life is very trivial and very boring, and you look for other people who think the same.
— seventeen-year-old girl, heroin addict

I started shooting heroin at the age of twelve and was a junkie till I was fifteen. I went cold turkey eight or nine times, but after each cold turkey I'd see my old friends again, and then I'd go back to heroin.
— nineteen-year-old girl, former heroin addict

smoking tobacco and marijuana even though they don't like their effects, only to feel accepted — in much the same way that they might adopt faddish styles of dress that do not suit them. Young people often see drugs as symbols of maturity and sophistication, and fear that if they do not use them they will be denied entry into in-crowds. Cigarette and alcohol advertising capitalize on these attitudes and fears.

Using drugs because "everybody else does it" probably isn't a very good reason, but it is certainly a very common one.

To establish an identity.   Often an individual or small group will take up the use of a prohibited substance or abuse a permitted one in order to feel special or create a sense of identity. Just as punk rockers wear outlandish clothes and make-up, some people adopt unusual or affected drug styles to get attention and recognition.

There are so many reasons why people might take drugs that it may be hard to say which ones are operating in any given instance. A person may take one drug for one reason and another for another reason, or take one drug for several reasons at once. Then again, people sometimes take drugs purely out of habit and not for any reason at all.

Suggested Reading

Andrew Weil's *The Natural Mind: A New Way of Looking at Drugs and the Higher Consciousness* (Boston: Houghton Mifflin, 1972) examines drug-taking as a method of changing consciousness and speculates on why altered states of consciousness are important to us.

Society and Drugs by Richard H. Blum and Associates (San Francisco: Jossey-Bass, 1970) is a good survey of drug use throughout history in various cultures.

In *The Joyous Cosmology: Adventures in the Chemistry of Consciousness* (New York: Vintage, 1965), philosopher Alan Watts gives a colorful picture of states of consciousness induced by hallucinogenic drugs. Watts experimented with these substances as an explorer of the mind and a searcher for religious experience.

Shaman Woman, Mainline Lady: Women's Writings on the Drug Experience, edited by Cynthia Palmer and Michael Horowitz (New York: William Morrow, 1982), is an anthology covering many times and cultures. It gives a broad overview of different ways of using many drugs.

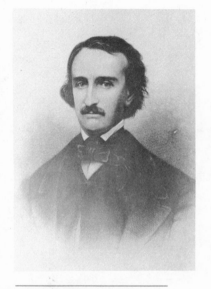

Edgar Allan Poe (1809–1849), the American writer and poet, was partial to laudanum (tincture of opium), and his macabre tales were no doubt influenced by his experiences with the drug. (Photo World/Free Lance Photographers Guild)

4

Relationships with Drugs

THE DESIRE TO CALL some drugs good and others bad has recently given rise to the term *drugs of abuse*. Government officials and medical doctors frequently talk about drugs of abuse, by which they usually mean all illegal substances. In their view, anyone using them is automatically guilty of drug abuse.

But what is drug abuse? To say that it is the use of a drug of abuse is circular and meaningless. We think that the use of *any* drug becomes abusive when it threatens a person's health or impairs social or economic functioning. Cigarette smokers with lung disease who continue to smoke are clearly abusing tobacco. Students who cannot concentrate on classroom activities because they are stoned are abusing marijuana. Alcoholics who are unable to hold down jobs are abusers of alcohol. Junkies who must steal to support their habits are abusers of heroin. On the other hand, any drug can be used in a nonabusive fashion, even if it is illegal or disapproved. There are many people who consume tobacco, marijuana, alcohol, and heroin without abusing them; that is, they remain healthy and fulfill their social and economic obligations. Drug abuse is not simply a matter of what drug a person chooses to consume; rather, it depends on the relationship an individual forms with that drug.

Many factors determine relationships with drugs. Obviously, the drug itself is one important factor; there is a whole science, pharmacology, devoted to finding out what drugs do.

Unfortunately, effects of drugs are difficult to specify. Different people show different responses to the same dose of the same drug, probably because people differ in biochemistry, just as they do in appearance. Even the same person may respond differently to the same dose of the same drug at different times. Pharmacologists attempt to minimize these variations by giving drugs to animals and people under controlled laboratory conditions. The results of these experiments enable them to classify drugs into different categories. For example, they can show most psychoactive drugs to be either stimulants or depressants of the nervous system.

Laboratory experiments also show us that the dose of a drug is a crucial variable. High doses of a substance may produce very different effects from low doses. Moderate doses of alcohol will give many people feelings of well-being and relaxation; high doses may cause incoordination, confusion, and sickness.

The way a drug is put into the body also shapes its effects. When you take a drug by mouth it enters the bloodstream slowly, and its influence on the nervous system is less intense than when you bypass the gastrointestinal tract by sniffing, smoking, or injecting it. High doses of drugs introduced by one of these more direct routes are likely to be more harmful and more addicting over time.

These pharmacological facts can explain some of the variations we see in the relationships people form with drugs. For instance, South American Indians who chew coca leaves swallow low doses of cocaine and do not seem to become abusers of that stimulant. People who put much larger doses of refined cocaine in their noses are much more likely to develop medical, social, and psychological problems. The abuse potential of snorting coke is far greater than the abuse potential of chewing coca. In other words, people are more likely to form good relationships with coca than with cocaine, and this difference clearly has some basis in pharmacology.

However, the laboratory is not the real world, and pharmacology can only explain certain aspects of human relationships with drugs. When people take drugs in the real world their experiences are often not what pharmacologists would predict. The reason is that outside the laboratory other factors can completely change the effects of drugs. One such factor is called *set;* set is what a person expects to happen when he or she takes a drug. Expectation is shaped by all of past experience — what a person has heard about the drug, read about it, seen of it, thought about it, and wants it to do. Sometimes it is not easy to

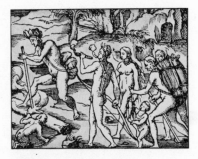

A Brazilian Indian smoking. From a French drawing dated 1558. (Fitz Hugh Ludlow Memorial Library)

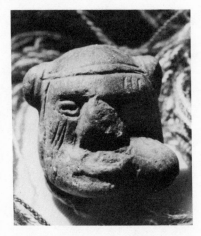

This carved stone head from Colombia shows a coca user, his cheek bulged out with leaves. It dates from about 1400. (Michael R. Aldrich)

find out what people expect of a drug because their real feelings might be hidden from themselves. A teen-age boy smoking marijuana for the first time may think he is eager to have a new experience, whereas unconsciously he may be terrified of losing his mind or getting so stoned he will never come down. Such unconscious fears can determine reactions to marijuana more than the actual effect of the drug.

Set can also be as important as pharmacology in shaping long-term relationships with drugs. For example, some people expect marijuana to make them relaxed and tired and so will use it only occasionally at bedtime to help fall asleep, whereas others, who feel that pot reduces their anxiety and makes it

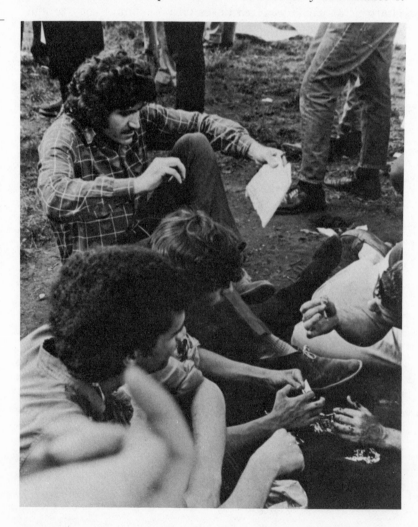

A "smoke-in" in Tompkins Square Park, New York City, 1968. (Shelly Rusten, Free Lance Photographers Guild)

easier to relate to people, use it so frequently throughout the day that they become dependent on it.

Setting is another factor that modifies pharmacology. Setting is the environment in which a drug is used — not just the physical environment but also the social and cultural environment. During the Vietnam War many American soldiers got into the habit of smoking large amounts of the high-grade heroin that was cheap and easily available to them in Southeast Asia. They rolled it into cigarettes with tobacco or marijuana and used it primarily to escape boredom, because for many American soldiers Vietnam was, more than anything else, boring, and because heroin seems to make time pass more quickly. Pharmacologists would have predicted that most of these soldiers would become heroin addicts, but in fact, most of them stopped using opiates as soon as they came home. It was the special setting of army life in Vietnam that shaped this pattern of drug use, and when people left that setting most of them stopped easily.

Set and setting together can modify pharmacology drastically. Therefore, talking about the effects of drugs in the real world is not so simple. Effects of drugs are relative to particular people, places, and times. In ancient India, marijuana was eaten for religious purposes; people used it for its effects on consciousness in socially accepted ways. In England and America during the nineteenth century, doctors gave tincture of marijuana to sick people as a remedy, and most patients never reported getting high on it, probably because they did not expect to and so ignored the psychoactive effects. In the United States in the 1920s, members of certain subcultures began smoking marijuana to feel high — a practice regarded as deviant by the dominant culture. Many early marijuana smokers freaked out and some even committed acts of violence under its influence. Today, the smoking of marijuana is accepted in many circles, and users think it decreases aggression and hostility.

The fact that effects of psychoactive drugs can change so much from person to person, from culture to culture, and from age to age points up the folly of calling any drug good or bad. But if there is no such thing as a drug of abuse, still there *is* drug abuse, and learning to recognize it is important. Only in analyzing people's relationships with drugs can *good* and *bad* have meaning. Some people may be upset by the notion that you can have a good relationship with a drug, but chances are they fail to acknowledge that many socially accepted substances are, in fact, drugs.

Good relationships with drugs have four common characteristics:

1. *Recognition that the substance you are using is a drug and awareness of what it does to your body.* People who wind up in the worst relationships with drugs often have little understanding of the substances they use. They think coffee is just a beverage, marijuana an herb, and diet pills just "appetite suppressants." *All drugs have the potential to cause trouble unless people take care not to let their use of them get out of control.* A necessary first step is to acknowledge the nature of the substances in use and to understand their effects.

2. *Experience of a useful effect of the drug over time.* People who begin to use drugs regularly often find that their early experiences with them are the best; as they use the drugs more and more frequently, the effects they like seem to diminish. People in the worst relationships with drugs often use them very heavily but get the least out of them. This curious pattern happens with all drugs and can be very frustrating. Frequency of use is the critical factor in determining whether the effect of a drug will last over time. If the experience you like from a drug begins to fade, that is a sign you are using too much too often. If you ignore the warning and continue consuming the drug at the same frequency, you will begin to slide into a worse and worse relationship with it.

3. *Ease of separation from use of the drug.* One of the more striking features of a bad relationship with a drug is dependence: it controls you more than you control it. People in good relationships with drugs can take them or leave them.*

4. *Freedom from adverse effects on health or behavior.* People vary in their susceptibility to the adverse effects of drugs. Some individuals can smoke cigarettes all their lives and never develop lung disease. Some people can snort cocaine frequently and remain physically and psychologically healthy and socially productive. Others cannot. Using drugs in ways that produce adverse effects on health and behavior and continuing their use in spite of these effects is the defining characteristic of drug abuse.

Whether a drug is legal or illegal, approved or disapproved, obtained from a physician or bought on the black market, if the user is aware of its nature, can maintain a useful effect from it

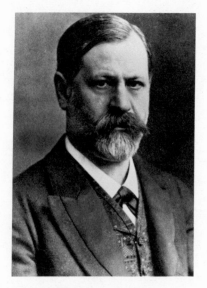

Sigmund Freud (1856–1939). The father of psychoanalysis, Freud was an early enthusiast for cocaine as well as an addicted cigar smoker (twenty a day). He later repudiated cocaine, but continued smoking for most of his life and died of a tobacco-related oral cancer. (National Library of Medicine. Courtesy of the New York Psychoanalytic Institute Archives)

*Dependence on drugs is discussed at length in Chapter 12.

over time, can easily separate himself or herself from it, and can remain free from adverse effects, that is a good relationship with the drug.

Bad relationships with drugs begin with ignorance of the nature of the substance and loss of the desired effect with increasing frequency of use, and progress to difficulty in leaving the drug alone, with eventual impairment of health or social functioning.

Any drug can be used successfully, no matter how bad its reputation, and any drug can be abused, no matter how accepted it is. There are no good or bad drugs; there are only good and bad relationships with drugs.

Suggested Reading

Few books on drugs make a clear distinction between use and abuse. One that does is *Our Chemical Culture: Drug Use and Misuse* by Marcia J. Summers et al. (Madison, Wisconsin: STASH Press, 1975); it is written for a high-school audience.

Drugs: A Multimedia Sourcebook for Young Adults by Sharon Ashenbrenner Charles and Sari Feldman (New York: Neal Schumann, 1980) is an annotated listing of books, pamphlets, and films, including works of fiction, and gives addresses for ordering these materials.

In *The Marriage of the Sun and Moon: A Quest for Unity in Consciousness* (Boston: Houghton Mifflin, 1980), Andrew Weil presents a number of case examples of substances and techniques that can make people high. Some involve drugs such as magic mushrooms, coca leaves, and marijuana; others do not — uncontrolled laughter, Indian sweat baths, eating mangoes and hot chilies, and watching eclipses of the sun, for example. The ways people think about these substances and activities determine the relationships formed with them.

5

Types of Drugs

PSYCHOACTIVE DRUGS can be classified according to
whether they are natural or manmade, produced
by our own bodies or by plants, crude mixtures of
substances or single, purified chemicals. These differences may influence the relationships people form
with drugs, and users, especially, should be aware of
them.

Endogenous (In-the-Body) Drugs

The human body, especially in the brain and certain glands,
makes powerful chemicals that affect our moods, thoughts, and
actions. We call these substances endogenous drugs, using a
term with Greek roots meaning "made within." Interestingly
enough, they resemble many of the external chemicals people
take to change their consciousness.

The discovery of endogenous drugs is a recent scientific
breakthrough. By 1950, brain researchers had come to understand that psychoactive drugs work by fitting into special receptor sites on nerve cells just as keys fit into locks. Only when a
drug molecule plugs into a receptor that fits it does it produce
an effect, such as causing a nerve cell to fire an electrical impulse or preventing it from firing one. This principle is the cor-
nerstone of current theory about drugs and the nervous system.

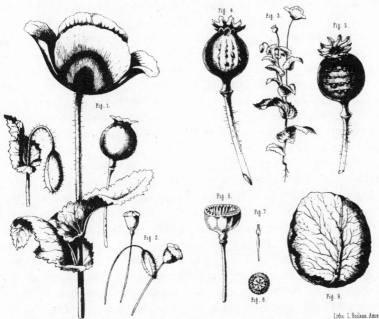

Litho. L. Boileau. Amiens

For example, pharmacologists learned that morphine and heroin attach to special opiate receptors on nerve cells in certain parts of the brain. But why should our brains have receptors designed to fit molecules made by poppy plants? Some researchers suggested that opiate receptors really exist for other substances made by the brain itself — molecules whose shapes happen to be similar to those of opiates. In 1975 this suggestion was confirmed with the discovery of a group of chemicals called endorphins. Endorphins are the brain's own narcotics, producing most of the effects of poppy drugs, including euphoria and reduction of pain.

Endorphins are now under intense investigation because they are likely to reveal much about the workings of our minds and bodies. People who have high tolerance for pain may produce more of these endogenous narcotics. When you wake up one day feeling high and unfazed by the problems that ordinarily get you down, your endorphin system might be in high gear. Some people may be born with an inability to make enough endorphins; possibly, they are the ones who find opiates especially pleasant and come to rely on them to cope with the pain and stress of day-to-day existence.

The discovery of endorphins also raises interesting questions. Why have the human brain and the poppy evolved chemi-

Old botanical drawing of an opium poppy, showing details of the unripe pods with incisions to permit the flow of opium. (Courtesy of the Harvard College Library)

cals with similar effects when they are so unlike each other? Is this fact a mere coincidence or does it suggest a deep relationship between people and plants that underlies the age-old inclination to experiment with vegetable drugs? And what does it say about the "naturalness" of taking drugs? It is possible that endorphins and other endogenous agents are the basis of all the highs people experience, whether obtained with drugs or without. People who get high by meditating or running, for example, may have found ways to stimulate the production or release of their own neurochemicals.

Not only does the body make its own narcotics, it also makes representatives of most of the other categories of drugs discussed in this book. It certainly makes its own uppers in the form of adrenaline and noradrenaline. It makes its own downers in the form of serotonin and GABA (gamma-amino-butyric acid), chemicals that slow down transmission in the central nervous system. Sex hormones can be powerful antidepressants, working better than anything so far concocted in a laboratory. Probably the body also makes its own psychedelics — most likely DMT (dimethyltryptamine) or a close relative of it — since the pineal gland, deep in the brain, secretes hormones with a very similar molecular structure.

Because the drugs our bodies make are designed to fit exactly into receptors on nerves, they are very powerful and efficient in producing their effects. Scientists are just beginning to learn about them and will certainly have much to say on the subject in years to come. It will be interesting to know how the use of external drugs affects the production of internal ones. Possibly, regular use of a drug from outside decreases or shuts off the manufacture of the corresponding endogenous substance, and so creates a chemical basis for dependence and addiction.

Natural Drugs

Crude Forms

Most psychoactive drugs come from plants, and there are hundreds of plants with psychoactive properties. People have put most of them to use in one part of the world or another at one time or another. Often drug plants taste bad, are weak, or have unwanted side effects. Traditional peoples who use these plants, such as Native Americans, have come up with clever ways of preparing and ingesting them to maximize the desired effects or make them easier to take. Traditional peoples do not tamper with the chemical composition of the plants, however. For example, South American Indians have found that drying coca leaves and mixing them with ashes or other alkalis increases their stimulant effect. They have also learned to make a powerful snuff from the resin of the virola tree (a DMT-containing plant) in order to take psychedelic trips. In a similar way, Old World natives learned to roast coffee beans and extract them with hot water to prepare a flavorful and stimulating beverage.

Crude plant drugs contain complex mixtures of chemicals, all of which contribute to the effect of the whole. Often more of one chemical will be present than of any other, and that one may account for the most dramatic effects of the plant. Cocaine is the main drug in coca leaves and is responsible for the numbness in the mouth and much of the stimulation that coca chewers like. In the same way, caffeine is the predominant constituent of coffee. Doctors and pharmacologists refer to these predominating chemicals as the "active principles" of the plants, which would be fine except that it implies all the other constituents are inactive and unimportant.

In the mid-1800s, scientists first began to identify the active principles of well-known drug plants. They soon succeeded in isolating many and making them available in pure form. Doctors quickly began to treat patients with these purified derivatives. Today, most doctors regard green medicinal plants as old-fashioned and unscientific; they rely instead on refined white powders derived from plants. Because pharmacologists have also lost interest in plants and study only isolated active principles, they know little about how whole plants differ in their effects from refined drugs.

The relationships people form with plants are different from those they form with white powders. Crude natural drugs tend to be less toxic, and users tend to stay in better relationships with them over time. One reason for this difference is that plants are dilute preparations, since the active principles are combined not only with other drugs but also with inert vegetable matter. Drug plants commonly contain less than 5 percent of an active principle. (Coca rarely has more than 0.5 percent cocaine.) By contrast, refined preparations may approach 100 percent purity.

In addition, crude plants usually go into the body through the mouth and stomach, whereas purified chemicals can be put into the bloodstream more directly, such as by snorting or injecting. Harmful effects, both immediate and long-term, are more likely to appear when people put drugs directly into their bloodstreams without giving their bodies a chance to process them.

Finally, the many other compounds in drug plants — often a single plant will contain twenty or more active components — may modify the active principles, making them safer or softening their harsher actions on the body. These safety factors and modifiers are lost when the active principles are isolated from the crude drugs that nature provides.

Natural drugs in whole plant form are the safest types of drugs. They always have lower potentials for abuse. If people choose to take drugs, they would be wise to use natural plant forms in order to give themselves the best chance of avoiding problems.

Refined Forms

Morphine, cocaine, and mescaline are all examples of drugs that occur in plants but are commonly available in refined form as white powders, sold both legally and illegally. Some of them, such as mescaline, can easily be synthesized in laboratories, but even when they are, we can still call them natural drugs because the molecules already exist in nature. Others, such as cocaine and morphine, have more complex molecular structures. Chemists can make them in laboratories, but it is not cost efficient to do so. All the cocaine and morphine on the black market and in pharmacies are extracted from coca leaves and opium poppies.

An illegal cocaine laboratory in Peru. Coca leaves are first soaked in a solvent to extract the drugs they contain. (Jake Myers)

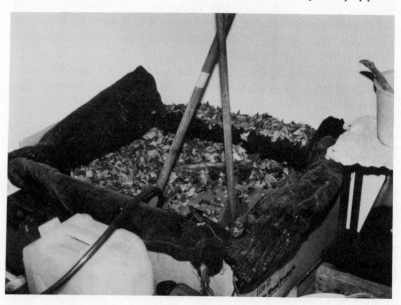

Extraction and purification of some plant drugs is long and complicated, requiring sophisticated techniques and equipment. In other cases the process is so simple that unskilled people can do it in kitchens. Black-market cocaine is usually made in primitive jungle factories; of course, it is likely to contain many impurities.

Whether natural drugs are manufactured by chemists or extracted from plants, they may be safer than drugs nature never thought of, because they interact more smoothly with the body's own chemistry. Since their structures tend to be closer to those of endogenous drugs, the effects of the two tend to be similar. As we have noted, however, it is important to distinguish between natural drugs in the dilute forms of crude plants and refined powders with much higher toxicity and abuse potential.

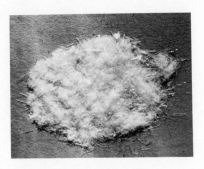

Mescaline crystals; 400 milligrams, a typical dose. (Jeremy Bigwood)

Semisynthetic Drugs

Pharmacologists often take refined natural drugs and change their chemical structures to vary their properties. A very simple change is to combine an insoluble drug from a plant with an acid to make a water-soluble salt. In this way the "freebase" form of cocaine, which is usually smoked because it will not dissolve, is turned into cocaine hydrochloride, a water-soluble compound that can be inhaled or injected.

A slightly more complicated transformation is the addition of chemical groups to a natural drug molecule to make it stronger. At the end of the nineteenth century, German chemists created aspirin by adding an acetic acid group to a natural pain-relieving chemical found in the bark of some willow trees. North American Indians drank willow-bark teas to treat headaches and rheumatism, but aspirin is a more powerful pain reliever than willow bark. (It is also much more toxic.) A similar addition of two acetic acid groups to morphine turns it into heroin, a similar but more potent drug. That is, it takes less heroin than morphine to produce the same effect.

These transformations of natural drugs result in new substances called semisynthetic drugs. Chemists like to make semisynthetic drugs because it is easier to play with an existing molecule than to start from scratch. Sometimes their experiments just intensify the actions of the original compounds, as in the examples of aspirin and heroin, while in other cases the results are completely novel. LSD (lysergic acid diethylamide) is an example of a semisynthetic drug with novel properties. It was made from a natural chemical in a fungus called ergot that attacks grasses and grains, but the original chemical (lysergic acid) is toxic and has little psychoactivity.

The ability of chemists to create new drugs from natural compounds raises an old argument about whether human beings should tamper with nature. We think people are meant to interact with the natural world and modify its creations. In fact, people can improve on nature. A fine example is the development of excellent varieties of fruits and vegetables from unimpressive wild species. The issue for us is whether the results of the manipulations are positive or negative. Plant selection and breeding that aim to enhance flavor and nutrition are clearly worthwhile. On the other hand, the production of square, hard, tasteless tomatoes to facilitate mass packing and shipping is inspired by greed for money rather than a desire to benefit humanity.

In the same way, when chemists tinker with natural drugs they should attempt to maximize desirable qualities. Extreme potency is not necessarily desirable, because it often goes hand in hand with great toxicity. We pay a high price today for our rejection of natural medicines in favor of potent chemicals. The tendency of pharmacologists and doctors to regard more potent drugs as more modern and more scientific encourages the use of dangerous derivatives of plants when often the milder, natural originals would do as well.

Synthetic Drugs

Wholly synthetic drugs are made from scratch in the laboratory and do not occur naturally. Valium, PCP (phencyclidine), and secobarbital (Seconal) are examples. It may be that synthetic drugs are the most dangerous of all and the hardest to form good relationships with, but it is risky to make such sweeping judgments. Very recently, researchers discovered Valium receptors in the human brain, making them think that the body must produce some internal analog to that completely synthetic tranquilizer. Did the chemists who created Valium in a laboratory just hit upon that molecule by chance? Has Valium become so popular because its effect resembles that of an endogenous substance? Or might Valium receptors have developed in the brain in response to use of the drug? It is interesting to speculate on these questions, even though science may never be able to answer them.

In the following pages we describe all the psychoactive drugs that people are likely to encounter, both those that are legal and those that are not. We discuss them category by category, explaining how they work and what their benefits and dangers are. In any category, such as stimulants, some drugs may be natural — in crude or refined form — some may be semisynthetic, and some totally synthetic. We do not dwell on these differences but encourage the reader to keep in mind that dilute, natural forms of substances are always safer and may give users the best chance to build stable relationships with the drugs they take.

Suggested Reading

There is no good book on the different types of drugs discussed in this chapter or on the new discoveries about endogenous drugs. An interesting book on the plant sources of natural drugs is William Emboden's *Narcotic Plants* (New York: Macmillan, 1979). Emboden is a botanist who uses the word *narcotic* as a synonym for *psychoactive*. The book covers all categories of psychoactive plants: depressants, stimulants, hallucinogens, and deliriants. It includes many illustrations and color plates and much information on the traditions and uses of these plants in all parts of the world.

Richard R. Lingeman's *Drugs from A to Z: A Dictionary* (New York: McGraw-Hill, 1969) is a good, readable reference book on psychoactive drugs. It includes brand names, slang terms, and general information on effects.

6

Stimulants

STIMULANTS ARE DRUGS that make people feel more alert and energetic by activating or exciting the nervous system. There are many stimulant drugs in current use; some are plants found in nature, others are chemicals made in the laboratory. These different drugs produce somewhat different effects, lasting for varying lengths of time, but all of them raise the energy level of the nervous system in roughly the same way.

The individual nerves in our bodies communicate with each other both electrically and chemically. A nerve impulse is an electric discharge that moves quickly along the fiber of a nerve cell. The fiber may end at a muscle, a gland, or another nerve cell, but there is always a tiny space between the end of the nerve fiber and the next cell. To bridge this gap, the nerve fiber releases small amounts of powerful chemicals called neurotransmitters that affect the next cell. Some neurotransmitters are strong stimulants that cause muscle cells to contract, gland cells to secrete, and other nerve cells to fire off electrical discharges. The most common stimulant neurotransmitter is a chemical called noradrenaline or norepinephrine. This chemical is closely related to the hormone adrenaline (or epinephrine), which is produced by our adrenal glands.*

Adrenal is a Latin word meaning "on the kidney," because the adrenal glands sit on top of the kidneys like little caps. *Epinephros* means the same thing in

Stimulant drugs work by causing nerve fibers to release noradrenaline and other stimulating neurotransmitters. Although different stimulants bring about this release in different ways, the end result is always the same: the release of more stimulating neurotransmitters. So, the stimulation people feel when they take stimulant drugs is simply a result of the body's own chemical energy going to work in the nervous system. The drug just makes the body expend it sooner and in greater quantity than it would ordinarily.

This release of chemical energy in the form of noradrenaline causes certain predictable changes in the mind and body. It makes a person feel wakeful, alert, and, often, happy. It makes the heart beat faster and may cause the blood pressure to rise. Because it produces changes in blood flow, the fingertips and tip of the nose may become cold. It gives a feeling of butterflies in the stomach and may cause a laxative effect.

Some of these changes are mediated by a branch of the nervous system called the sympathetic nervous system. The main function of the sympathetic nervous system is to respond to emergencies by preparing the body for fight or flight. It does so by shutting down nonessential functions and speeding up vital ones. The sympathetic nervous system relies on noradrenaline as its chemical messenger.

Now, noradrenaline acts in many of the same ways as adrenaline, the hormone secreted by the adrenal glands, also in response to emergencies. Experiences that cause the adrenals to secrete adrenaline into the bloodstream produce feelings very much like those of stimulant drugs. The rush of excitement one gets on a roller coaster ride, for example, may feel a lot like the effect of a dose of amphetamine, and no doubt both these techniques are popular for the same reason — because they give people a sense of increased mental and physical energy, and make them feel, temporarily at least, more alive.

In recent years scientists have begun to find out many interesting things about biorhythms, the cycles by which our vital processes wax and wane. The most obvious daily biorhythm is that of sleeping and waking. Production of hormones and neurotransmitters has its own ups and downs, and these cycles probably explain why people feel naturally stimulated at certain times and naturally lethargic at others. A common pattern is to

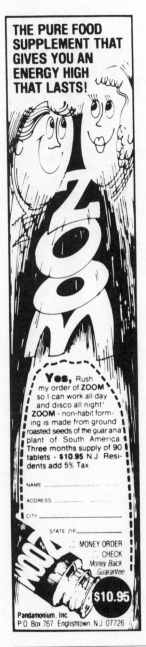

(Courtesy of Pandamonium, Inc.)

Greek. In America the Parke-Davis pharmaceutical company succeeded in registering Adrenalin as a trademark for its brand of adrenal hormone, and as a result American scientists generally use the more cumbersome words *epinephrine* and *norepinephrine*. We prefer the Latin form.

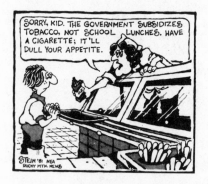

SORRY, KID. THE GOVERNMENT SUBSIDIZES TOBACCO, NOT SCHOOL LUNCHES. HAVE A CIGARETTE; IT'LL DULL YOUR APPETITE.

STEIN '81 NEA
ROCKY MTN. NEWS

(Reprinted from the *Rocky Mountain News*, Denver, Colorado)

feel energetic and able to concentrate well in the morning but to become tired and mentally sluggish in the late afternoon.

One reason that stimulant drugs are popular is that they give temporary control over rhythms of wakefulness and the ups and downs of mood. If you have a mental task to do at 3 P.M., when your brain wants to rest, you can mobilize it to concentrate by taking a stimulant drug and thereby forcing your nervous system to release some of its stored-up chemical energy. Or if you have to drive a long distance at night when your whole nervous system is ready for sleep, you can stay awake by putting a stimulant into your body. Or if you are feeling depressed when you have to go out and meet important people, a stimulant might brighten your mood for a while.

Another reason people like stimulants is that they suppress hunger, making it possible to think about something other than food and concentrate better on the task at hand. Not eating, moreover, tends to further increase one's energy and sense of alertness. The reason stimulant drugs suppress hunger probably has to do with the preparation of the body for emergencies. In emergencies, all digestive functions become nonessential compared to such processes as blood circulation and speed of muscular response. Under stress, therefore, the body shifts energy away from the stomach and intestines to the brain, heart, and blood vessels.

Because the nerves and muscles receive more attention under the effect of stimulants, these drugs may improve certain kinds of physical and mental performance for a time. They may enable people to concentrate longer and better or to perform physical work more efficiently and with greater endurance. This probably explains why these drugs are especially popular with students and athletes.

Of course, not everyone is affected by stimulants in the same way; some people find their effects unpleasant, just as some people find roller coaster rides unpleasant. Far from making everyone cheerful and alert, these drugs make many people anxious, jittery, and unable to sit still. Some people are so sensitive to stimulants that they cannot sleep at all even twelve hours after taking a small dose. Others get such distressing symptoms as heart palpitations, diarrhea, and urinary frequency. Instead of automatically improving physical and mental performance, stimulants sometimes just make people do poor work faster. There are famous stories of college students who wrote what they imagined to be brilliant final exams under the influence of amphetamines, only to find later that they had written the same line over and over or scribbled the whole exam on one illegible page.

Still, at first glance, stimulants sound attractive: they can make you feel alert, happy, wakeful, energetic, strong, and resistant to hunger, boredom, and fatigue. But one of life's basic rules is, You Never Get Something for Nothing (or, There's No Such Thing as a Free Lunch), and stimulants are no exception to this rule.

The most serious problems with stimulant drugs result from the way they work. For, instead of miraculously delivering free gifts of cosmic energy, stimulants merely force the body to give up some of its own energy reserves. So when the effect of a stimulant wears off, the body is left with less energy than usual and must replenish its supplies.

People experience this depletion of energy as a "down" or "low" state, marked by the very same feelings they take stimulants to avoid: namely, sleepiness, lethargy, laziness, mental fatigue, and depression. The price you pay for the good feeling a stimulant gives you is a not-so-good feeling when the stimulant wears off.

Now, if you are willing to pay this price and let the body recharge itself, there is nothing wrong with using stimulants now and then. The trouble is that many people are not willing to let their bodies readjust; they want to feel good again right away, so they take another dose of the drug. It's very easy to fall into a pattern of using stimulants all the time in order to avoid the down feeling that follows the initial up.

Unfortunately, when they are used in this way, stimulants quickly produce dependence. People who take stimulants regularly find they cannot function normally without them. They need them just to open their eyes in the morning, move their bowels, work, or do any of the tasks of everyday life. Without them they just don't feel like doing much of anything.

Kinds of Stimulants

Coffee and Other Caffeine-Containing Plants
Caffeine, the most popular natural stimulant, is found in a number of plants throughout the world. The drug was first isolated from coffee in 1821 and was named for that plant, but the effects of coffee and caffeine differ. In many ways coffee seems to be more powerful than refined caffeine or other caffeine-containing plants.

In the morning I drink two cups of coffee. If I don't, I feel irritable. If I drink three cups, I get a little speedy, but with two I feel just about right.
— thirty-nine-year-old man, college administrator

Far beyond all other pleasures, rarer than jewels or treasures, sweeter than grape from the vine. Yes! Yes! Greatest of pleasures! Coffee, coffee, how I love its flavor, and if you would win my favor, yes! Yes! let me have coffee, let me have my coffee strong.
— from the Coffee Cantata, by Johann Sebastian Bach (1685–1750)

A shrubby tree native to Ethiopia, coffee is now cultivated in many tropical countries throughout the world. Its bright red fruits, called cherries, each contain two seeds, or beans. The raw beans are gray-green and odorless, but when roasted they turn dark brown and develop their characteristic aroma and flavor. Legend has it that coffee was first discovered long ago by Ethiopian nomads who noticed that their domestic animals became frisky after eating the fruits of the trees. When people tried eating the seeds, they got frisky too, and eventually they learned to make a flavorful drink from the roasted seeds.

More than a thousand years ago, groups of Muslims in the Middle East began using coffee in religious rituals and ceremonies. Groups of men would meet one night a week, drink large amounts of coffee, and stay up all night praying and chanting. These mystics confined their use of coffee to occasional ceremonies, but as coffee became more widely known, other people began to use it, not for religious reasons but just because they liked its stimulant effect. When people started to drink coffee every day in large amounts, many of them found they couldn't stop.

When it first came to Europe in the seventeenth century,

Lloyd's Coffee House, London, about 1698. Lloyd's of London was born here and with it the modern insurance industry. (The Bettman Archive, Inc.)

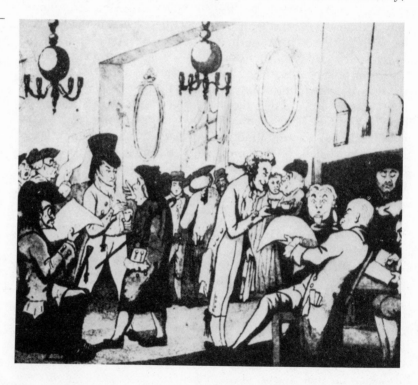

coffee stirred up great opposition as a new and unapproved drug. Authorities tried to prohibit its use, but of course their efforts were to no avail; coffee soon established itself there and all over the world. Coffee houses sprang up in all European cities, and whole populations became dependent on the drug almost overnight. Johann Sebastian Bach is rumored to have been a coffee addict. He extolled the virtues of the new drink in his famous Coffee Cantata. The French writer Balzac could not work without coffee. He drank larger and larger amounts of brews so strong they looked like thick soup, then complained of the stomach cramps they gave him.

Today coffee is a thoroughly approved drug — so approved, in fact, that many people who drink it regularly are surprised to learn it is a drug at all, let alone a powerful drug that can cause dependence and illness.

The truth is that coffee is a strong stimulant, one that is hard on certain parts of the body. It is irritating to the stomach, for example, and many people who drink a lot of it have indigestion most of the time. (In the United States, where coffee is regularly consumed in large quantities, there are nearly as many brands of antacids as there are brands of coffee.) It is irritating to the bladder, too, especially in women, and is a frequent cause of urinary complaints. Coffee also makes many people shaky by upsetting the delicate balance between nerves and muscles.

Today dependence on coffee is very common in Western society. Many regular users cannot think clearly in the morning until they have had their first cup. Without it they can't concentrate, move their bowels, or do their work. Also, they suffer real withdrawal symptoms — severe headaches, for example — if they stop using coffee suddenly. Such problems all come from using coffee too frequently so that the body never gets a chance to replenish its stores of chemical energy and comes to rely more and more on the external drug.

Coffee and caffeine have been accused of causing birth defects. There is no agreement on this possibility among scientists, but pregnant women should remember that coffee and caffeine are drugs and should not consume them in large amounts. Recently, medical researchers have found evidence linking coffee (but not other caffeine drinks) with cancer of the pancreas, an untreatable form of cancer that has been on the increase among Americans. The evidence is still weak, however, so it would be premature to give up occasional cups of coffee for fear of developing this disease. Coffee drinkers should watch for further information on this possible health risk.

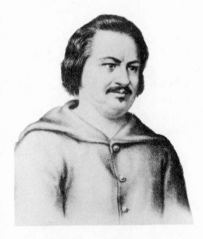

Honoré de Balzac (1799–1850), the great French writer, was also a great coffee addict. (Paul Thompson, Photo World/Free Lance Photographers Guild)

We had a kettle; we let it leak.
Our not repairing it made it
*   worse.*
We haven't had any tea for a
*   week . . .*
The bottom is out of the
*   Universe.*
— "Natural Theology," by
Rudyard Kipling (1865–1936)

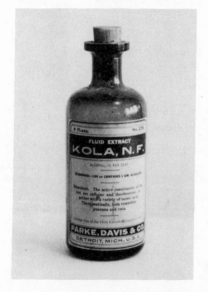

An extract of cola nut in alcohol formerly was used in medicine. The label of this old bottle reads, "Therapeutically, kola resembles guaraná and coca." (Michael R. Aldrich)

Other caffeine beverages don't seem to be as powerful or as toxic as coffee — even though they may contain as much caffeine or equivalent drugs. Tea is not nearly so irritating to the body as coffee, and cases of dependence on tea are less common. This is probably because coffee contains other substances that, by adding to the effect of the caffeine, make it a stronger drug. (Pharmacologists call this kind of interaction synergism.)

Of course, tea is a stimulant, and if you drink it in large amounts or make it strong enough, you can get powerful effects, including jitteriness and insomnia. In England, tea drinking has been a national pastime and habit ever since the early seventeenth century, when it was introduced from the Orient. In Japan, the tea ceremony is a very elaborate ritual built around the consumption of a special green tea powder that is whipped with water into a bitter, frothy drink.

Cola is a caffeine-containing seed, or nut, from a tropical tree, the cola tree. In some African countries cola nuts are so valuable they are used as money. The nuts have a bitter, aromatic taste, and people chew them for their stimulating effect. Bottled cola drinks have very little cola nut in them and do not taste like cola nuts at all. Though they do contain caffeine, it is usually synthetic caffeine or caffeine extracted from coffee or tea. These soft drinks are also drugs, and people can become dependent on them, as with coffee. Also, they contain a lot of sugar.

The combination of sugar and caffeine seems to be especially habit-forming. Many people drink enormous amounts of cola, and though they may think they are merely quenching their thirst, they are also consuming calories, enough sugar to damage their teeth (and possibly upset their metabolism), not to mention large doses of caffeine. Like other stimulants, cola drinks are not unhealthy if used in moderation; people who like them should just be aware of their nature and their potential for abuse.*

In other parts of the world, people use a number of less well known caffeine plants. The national drink of Brazil is guaraná (pronounced gwah-rah-NAH), made from the seeds of a jungle shrub. It contains more caffeine than coffee and is often made into sweet, carbonated drinks. Recently, tablets of guaraná powder have appeared in health food stores in the United States under such brand names as ZOOM and ZING. These are being

*The popularity of stimulating cola drinks has led manufacturers to add caffeine to some other flavors of carbonated beverages. Drinks so fortified must list caffeine as an ingredient. If you do not want to take drugs with your soda, you should make a habit of reading the information on bottles and cans.

marketed as new organic stimulants from the Amazon jungle.

In Argentina the most popular caffeine drink is maté (pronounced mah-TAY), which is made from the leaves of a holly plant. Some kinds of maté taste like smoky tea. Maté leaves can be bought in most health food stores and are ingredients in some herbal tea mixtures, such as Celestial Seasonings' Morning Thunder.

One of the most famous sources of caffeine is chocolate, also made from the seeds of a tropical tree.* Chocolate, which con-

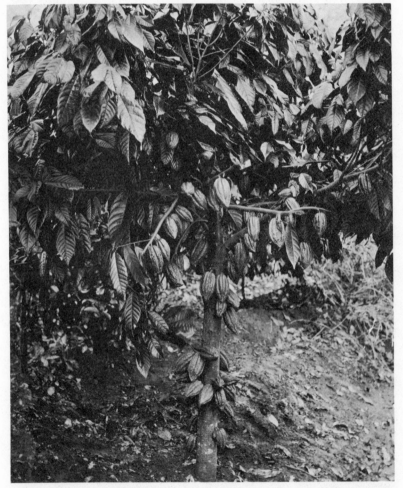

*The tree is called cacao (pronounced cah-COW), and its seeds are cacao beans, or cocoa beans. The fat in them is cocoa butter. White chocolate is just cocoa butter mixed with sugar. The roasted, ground-up beans, with most of the fat removed, are cocoa. Regular chocolate is made by adding extra fat to roasted, ground-up beans.

Five years ago, hoping to kick a chocolate habit that was significantly affecting my life, I enrolled in a program at the Shick Center for the Control of Smoking, Alcoholism, and Overeating, in Los Angeles. I was then thirty-three. I could not remember the last time I had managed to get through a whole day without eating chocolate in one form or another, usually in quantities most people would regard as excessive, if not appalling . . . Frankly, I am mystified by what happened and to this day cannot explain it. Being addicted to chocolate was so much a part of my definition of myself that it constantly amazes me to think that I am now free of it.
— thirty-eight-year-old woman, social worker

A cacao tree, source of chocolate and cocoa. The pods grow directly from the trunk and branches. (Harvard Botanical Museum)

tains a lot of fat and is very bitter, must be mixed with sugar to make it palatable. It, too, contains a stimulating drug, and cases of chocolate dependence are easy to find. You probably know a few "chocolate freaks." People who regularly consume chocolate or go on chocolate-eating binges may not realize they are involved with a drug, but their consumption usually follows the same sort of pattern as with coffee, tea, and cola drinks. (Do you know any vanilla freaks or butterscotch freaks?)

Cacao was known to the ancient Aztecs, who considered it a sacred plant and used it in religious rituals. In moderation chocolate is a pleasant and interesting addition to the diet, but overuse is not wise, especially since the combination of sugar, fat, and drugs can be so habit-forming. People who tend to gain weight easily should be especially careful about their intake of chocolate.

Coca and Cocaine

Coca, a shrub native to the hot, humid valleys of the eastern slopes of the Andes, has been cultivated by the Indians of South America for thousands of years. Today the plant is legal in Peru and Bolivia, where millions of Indians still chew coca leaves every day as a stimulant and medicine. (Coca, by the way, is not related to cocoa.)

Indian women in Peru sorting coca leaves. (Timothy Plowman)

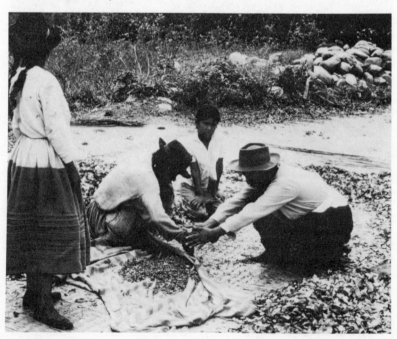

Coca contains fourteen drugs, cocaine being the most important. The other drugs are present in smaller amounts and seem to modify the stimulating effect of the cocaine. In addition, coca leaves contain many vitamins and minerals that are probably important in the diets of Indians who use them. There are several varieties of coca: some taste like green tea, some like wintergreen. Coca users put dried leaves in the mouth and work them into a large wad. They suck on this wad for thirty minutes or so, swallowing the juices, after which they spit out the residue. To get an effect from coca, a tiny amount of some alkali, such as lime (the powdered mineral) or ashes, must be added to the wad of leaves.

After a few minutes of chewing coca, the mouth and tongue become numb; then people begin to experience the usual effects of stimulants. Unlike coffee, coca soothes the stomach and doesn't produce jitteriness. It may also be more powerful than caffeine in producing a good mood.

In the late 1800s coca became very popular in Europe and America in the form of tonics and wines. Coca-Cola began as one of these early preparations. At the same time, scientists isolated cocaine from the leaves and made it available to doctors in the form of a pure white powder. As the first local anesthetic, cocaine revolutionized surgery, especially eye operations, which had always been terribly painful and difficult. In the 1880s doctors began to prescribe cocaine for all sorts of medical problems, including dependence on opiates and alcohol. It soon became apparent that this kind of treatment was not a good idea, because many patients suffered ill effects from cocaine, and many became dependent on it. So, in the early 1900s, laws were passed against the widespread use of coca and cocaine. The Coca-Cola Company took cocaine out of its drink (it still contains a drug-free extract of the leaves as a flavor). Other coca products swiftly disappeared from the shelves of drugstores. Safer local anesthetics were invented in laboratories, and today doctors use cocaine only for certain operations in the eye, nose, throat, and mouth.

Since then, a huge black market has developed to supply cocaine to the many people who like the feeling it gives. All illegal cocaine comes from leaves grown and processed in South America. It is always cut (diluted) with various substances before reaching consumers here. Most people snort cocaine; that is, they snuff the powder up their noses. Used in this way, the stimulant effects come on very fast, are very intense, and are very short-lived. Some people shoot cocaine, that is, inject it

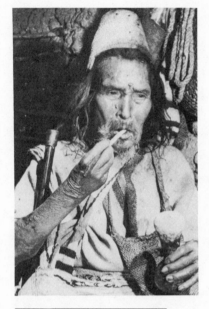

Colombian Indian coca chewer. He adds powdered lime to the wad of leaves in his mouth by moistening a stick, dipping it in the lime container in his other hand, then rubbing the white powder on the leaves. (Michael R. Aldrich)

intravenously,* which gives even faster, more intense, and shorter effects; and some people smoke a special form of cocaine called freebase in water pipes. Freebasing has become popular recently. It puts cocaine into the bloodstream even faster than intravenous injection and gives similar effects — very intense and very brief. Few people take cocaine by mouth, even though it works and is actually much safer that way.

Coca and cocaine are very different, and the difference shows how it is easier to form good relationships with natural drugs than with isolated and refined ones.

Coca leaves contain low concentrations of cocaine (usually only 0.5 percent), in combination with other drugs that modify its effects in a good way, and with valuable nutrients. The cocaine is highly diluted by inactive leaf material. What's more, getting stimulation from coca takes work: you have to chew a mouthful of leaves for half an hour. In this natural form, small amounts of cocaine enter the bloodstream slowly through the mouth and stomach.

Relatively pure street cocaine may contain 60 percent of the drug, which, when it is put directly into the nose, lungs, or veins, enters the bloodstream all at once. The stimulation, or "rush," is therefore very intense, but it lasts only a short time, usually disappearing within fifteen minutes to a half-hour. Then the user may feel down: tired, sluggish, unhappy. Because cocaine can make people feel so good for so short a time and not so good immediately thereafter, users tend to go on using it, trying to get back the good feeling. Many people can't leave this drug alone if they have it, even though all they get from it after a while are the unpleasant effects characteristic of all stimulants used in excess: anxiety, insomnia, and general feelings of discomfort. Besides, snorting too much cocaine leads to irritation of the nose, while smoking it may be bad for the lungs and is even more likely to lead to overuse and a stubborn habit.

Indians in South America, on the other hand, rarely have any problems with coca leaf. They can take it or leave it, continue to get good effects from it over time, and use the stimulation to help them work or socialize. They also use it as a medicine for a variety of illnesses, especially digestive ones. Among South American Indians there is little abuse of coca leaf.

In recent years, cocaine has become very fashionable in the United States. It is now very expensive, costing upwards of $100 a gram or $2000 an ounce. (The smokable freebase form is even

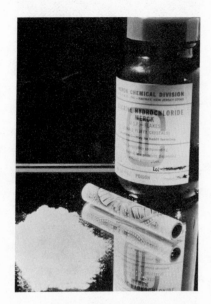

When cocaine hydrochloride was first isolated in the late 1880s it revolutionized surgery and was widely prescribed for a time. Now, in the 1980s, its medical application is limited, but its popularity as a recreational drug is growing by leaps and bounds. On the black market, this ounce of pure, pharmaceutical cocaine would be worth upwards of $2000. (Jeremy Bigwood)

---

*The health problems of intravenous drug use are discussed in Chapter 12.

more costly.) A few people can easily go through a gram of cocaine in a single evening, and heavy users may develop habits costing $15,000 a year and more. Occasional snorting of cocaine in social situations is probably not harmful, but one should be aware that the possibility of using this stimulant in excess is very real, and that abuse of cocaine can have ill effects on physical and emotional health as well as on productivity.

It seems a shame that the laws and policies on drugs in our society have led to the disappearance of coca along with knowledge of its uses and benefits. At the same time, by outlawing something that many people want, they have made it profitable to smuggle the concentrated drug, and so have encouraged the growth of a vast black market in cocaine.

Amphetamines and Related Drugs

Amphetamines are synthetic stimulants that were invented in Germany in the 1930s. Their chemical structures resemble those of adrenaline and noradrenaline, the body's own stimulants. Their effects resemble those of cocaine but are much longer lasting. A single oral dose of amphetamine usually stimulates the body for at least four hours.

Amphetamines are more toxic than cocaine and, when abused, cause worse problems. The body has a great capacity to metabolize and eliminate cocaine: the liver can detoxify a lethal dose of cocaine every thirty minutes. It cannot handle amphetamines as efficiently. At the same time, people can establish stable relationships with amphetamines more easily than they can with cocaine, probably because the intensely pleasureful but very short effect of cocaine is more seductive and invites repetitive dosing.

For many years after their invention, amphetamines were tolerated and their use was even encouraged by authorities. Soldiers in World War II received rations of amphetamines to make them march longer and fight better. The governments of several countries, among them the Soviet Union, experimented with giving amphetamines to factory workers, hoping to make them more productive (which, in the long run, they failed to do). Doctors in this country have prescribed them in great quantity for even more questionable reasons.

In the 1950s and 1960s, the U.S. pharmaceutical industry manufactured enormous quantities of amphetamines, many of which turned up on the black market. The companies urged doctors to prescribe their products for depressed housewives and people with weight problems.

I decided to try and make up for lost time by staying up all night to study for my European history exam, but by midnight the text was blurring before my eyes . . . An upperclassman took pity on me and offered me a green-and-white capsule along with the promise that my drowsiness would be cured by taking it. I took it without a second thought, and within half an hour or so found myself studying like mad. Not only was I completely engrossed in European history, I felt exhilarated; I was actually enjoying myself . . . I got an A on my history exam — as I was sure I had — and have been involved, to some extent, with amphetamines ever since.
— forty-two-year-old woman, writer

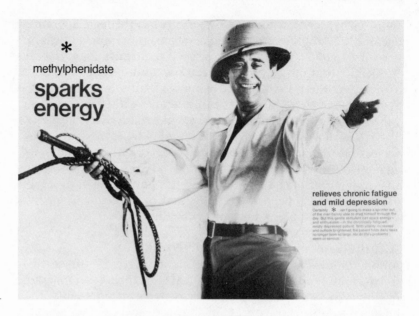

During the days of unrestricted prescription of amphetamine and amphetaminelike stimulants, pharmaceutical companies did not hesitate to suggest that these drugs made people happy and productive.

There are a number of different amphetamines, but all have the same basic effect. Plain amphetamine (Benzedrine) was the first to become popular. Dextroamphetamine (Dexedrine) and methamphetamine (Methedrine) are effective in lower doses but otherwise are similar to the parent compound. A few other drugs — methylphenidate (Ritalin), for example — resemble amphetamines in effect even though they have a different chemical structure.

Today we know that regular use of amphetamines, especially by people who are neurotic, depressed, or fat, is not a good idea. Not only do the drugs fail to help their problems, they often complicate matters by creating another kind of dependence. Most of the cases of amphetamine abuse in the past thirty years have involved legally manufactured and prescribed drugs. Beginning in the 1970s, criticism of the promotional practices of pharmaceutical companies and of the prescribing practices of physicians brought about severe restrictions on the medical use of these compounds. Today amphetamines can be prescribed for only a few conditions.

One of the more controversial uses still permitted is the control of hyperactivity in young children. For unknown reasons, amphetamines (and other stimulants) have calming effects on young children. Unfortunately, the diagnosis of hyperactivity often falls on children who simply misbehave or don't pay attention in school. Giving them amphetamines not only fails to get to the root of the problem, it introduces young people to powerful drugs and encourages among grownups the false notion that all of life's problems can be solved by taking pills.

As legal supplies and uses of amphetamines dwindled, black markets in them grew, and as so often happens, this change promoted abuse. In the days of legal pills, most users took them by mouth. Today many people snort powdered amphetamines in the same way as cocaine, and some even inject them intravenously.

Intravenous use of amphetamines first appeared in the late 1960s. Young "speed freaks" who fell into this pattern of use experienced very bad effects on their bodies and minds. After only a few weeks, they became emaciated and generally unhealthy; they stayed up for days on end, then "crashed" into stupors. They became jumpy, paranoid, and even psychotic. The drug subculture itself, realizing the dangers of shooting amphetamines, warned people about it with the phrase "speed kills."

A number of people find amphetamines useful for specific purposes. For example, some college students use them to study for or take exams. Some writers take them to work. Truckers and other drivers sometimes take them for long-distance travel on highways, especially at night. Athletes, such as football players, sometimes use them to play big games. Actors and dancers take them occasionally to perform. Used in this way — that is, taken by mouth on occasion for specific purposes or projects — amphetamines do not usually cause problems, especially if people rest afterward. Problems arise when people take amphetamines all the time, just because they like the feeling of stimulation.

"Look-Alike" Drugs

As both legal and illegal sources of amphetamines have dried up, a flood of bogus products has appeared. Called look-alikes, they are tablets and capsules made to look like pharmaceutical amphetamines but contain no controlled substances. Some are legally manufactured for over-the-counter sale in drugstores; others appear in head shops or are sold by mail order or on the street.

Look-alikes contain caffeine, ephedrine, or phenylpropanolamine, either singly or in combination. Ephedrine is a natural stimulant with a chemical structure resembling adrenaline that produces more anxiety and less euphoria than amphetamines. It occurs in a desert shrub and is used as a treatment for asthma.* Phenylpropanolamine is a synthetic drug that is

*See page 55.

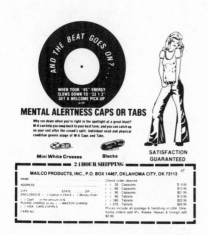

This ad for look-alike stimulants appeared in the magazine *High Times*. "White crosses" and "blacks" are slang terms for tablets and capsules of amphetamines.

Several years ago, I fell madly in love with an ex-smoker, a man who, though broad-minded in other respects, was a fanatic on the subject of cigarettes . . . I had always thought I'd be able to kick my addiction to cigarettes for someone I loved. That assumption turned out to be wrong. In the end, when forced to choose between love and cigarettes, I chose cigarettes. It was that simple. I did make one resolution at the time, which I have stuck to ever since. It was that I would never again become involved with a man who does not smoke cigarettes.
— forty-one-year-old woman, teacher

added to many cold remedies as a nasal decongestant. Recently, it has appeared in a number of over-the-counter diet pills, and although the manufacturers of these products claim it is not a stimulant, it is.

Look-alike drugs have received much bad publicity. They are accused of killing some people by causing strokes and disturbances of heartbeat. People with high blood pressure or histories of heart irregularities should be wary of them (as they should be of all stimulants). Since caffeine and ephedrine are generally considered safe after many years of use, phenyl-propanolamine is more likely to account for any toxicity of look-alike stimulants. Although it is currently authorized for inclusion in many over-the-counter compounds, its risks may be underestimated, especially when it is combined with caffeine and ephedrine or taken in high doses. (People who like amphetamines usually find the effects of look-alikes disappointing and so tend to take higher than recommended doses in an effort to feel more stimulation and euphoria.)

Another drawback of look-alikes is their cost: they are a very expensive way to buy the drugs they provide.

Tobacco and Nicotine

Tobacco is one of the most powerful stimulant plants known, and nicotine — its active principle — is one of the most toxic of all drugs. An average cigar contains enough nicotine to kill several people.

When tobacco is smoked, most of the nicotine is destroyed by the heat of burning. (To kill people with a cigar, you'd have to soak the cigar in water till it turned dark, then make people drink the liquid.) Nicotine is so strong and dangerous that the body very quickly develops tolerance to it to protect itself. If a person begins smoking regularly, tolerance to the poisonous effects of nicotine develops in a matter of hours (as compared to days or weeks for heroin and months for alcohol).

In the form of cigarettes, tobacco is the most addictive drug known. It is harder to break the habit of smoking cigarettes than it is to stop using heroin or alcohol. Moreover, many people learn to use alcohol and heroin in nonaddictive ways, whereas very few cigarette smokers can avoid becoming addicts. Occasionally, you will meet someone who smokes two or three cigarettes a day or even two or three a week, but such people are rare. Interestingly enough, these occasional users get high from smoking and like the effect, while most addicted smokers do not experience major changes in consciousness.

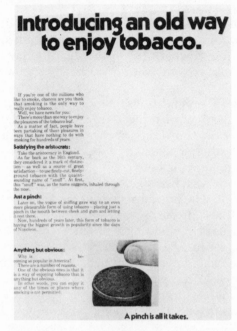

Introducing an old way to enjoy tobacco.

If you're one of the millions who like to smoke, chances are you think that smoking is the only way to really enjoy tobacco.

Well, we have news for you:

There's more than one way to enjoy the pleasures of the tobacco leaf.

As a matter of fact, people have been partaking of these pleasures in ways that have nothing to do with smoking for hundreds of years.

Satisfying the aristocrats:

Take the aristocracy in England.

As far back as the 16th century, they considered it a mark of distinction — as well as a source of great satisfaction — to use finely-cut, finely-ground tobacco with the quaint-sounding name of "snuff". At first, this "snuff" was, as the name suggests, inhaled through the nose.

Just a pinch:

Later on, the vogue of sniffing gave way to an even more pleasurable form of using tobacco — placing just a pinch in the mouth between cheek and gum and letting it rest there.

Now, hundreds of years later, this form of tobacco is having the biggest growth in popularity since the days of Napoleon.

Anything but obvious:

Why is it becoming so popular in America?

There are a number of reasons.

One of the obvious ones is that it is a way of enjoying tobacco that is anything but obvious.

In other words, you can enjoy it any of the times or places where smoking is not permitted.

A pinch is all it takes.

Smoke from cigarettes inhaled deeply delivers concentrated nicotine to vital brain centers within a few seconds — faster than heroin reaches the brain when it is injected into a vein in the arm. This fact probably explains why tobacco in the form of cigarettes is so addictive.

Doctors know also that regular cigarette smoking is a leading cause of serious disease of the lungs, heart, and blood vessels. This does not mean that everyone who smokes will necessarily get lung cancer. Some people smoke heavily all their lives and show no ill effects, probably because they have healthy lungs and strong constitutions to begin with. Others are not so lucky.

Pipes and cigars are less hazardous than cigarettes because smoke from them is harsher, discouraging deep inhalation. Many smokers of pipes and cigars do not inhale at all and so completely avoid the risk of lung disease. In addition, since they don't deliver rapid pulses of nicotine to their brains, they are less likely than cigarette smokers to become addicted to tobacco so strongly or so fast. Pipes and cigars are not without risk, however. They still put nicotine into the body, affecting the heart and circulation, and also increase the risk of cancer of the lips, mouth, and throat.

Some tobacco users take the drug without burning it. Tobacco chewers place wads of it in the mouth, letting the nicotine

Here is the way one large tobacco company recommends its plain and flavored snuffs. There is no mention that tobacco in this form is both less addicting and more stimulating. The main selling point is that you can use it undetected and in places where smoking is not permitted.

diffuse into their systems through blood vessels in the tongue and cheeks. Others use snuff (finely powdered tobacco) by inhaling it or putting pinches of it in the mouth. Many Amazonian Indians cook tobacco and water to form a paste that they rub on their gums.

All of these preparations give strong stimulation in the form of high doses of nicotine — higher than cigarettes, pipes, and cigars, because burning destroys so much of the nicotine in tobacco. Nevertheless, chewing tobacco or taking snuff is less addicting than smoking because it puts nicotine into the blood and brain much less directly.

Most people who put tobacco into the mouth or nose for the first time dislike it. It burns, tastes terrible, causes intense salivation and sneezing, and often produces rapid dizziness and nausea. With repeated trials, however, users grow tolerant to the worst effects and come to like the sensations in the mouth and nose. Tobacco companies now sell snuff as "smokeless tobacco," some of it with mint and fruit flavoring to make it more acceptable to novices. They promote it as a new and pleasant

The female and male cigarette addicts, as depicted by two of the major tobacco companies.

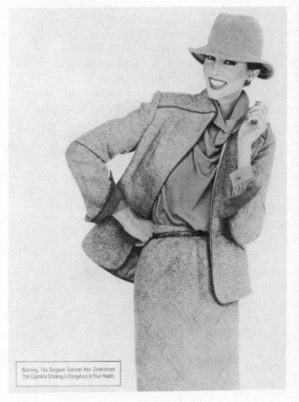

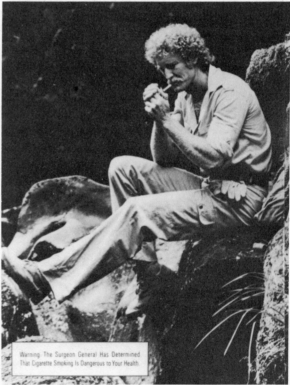

way to use the drug even in nonsmoking areas. Smokeless tobaccos have recently become popular among teen-agers, probably because it is easier to use the drug without detection. An unquestionable plus for snuff and chewing tobacco is that they do not pollute the air with smoke and expose nonusers to nicotine and other irritants.

Despite its toxicity and addictiveness, tobacco is a fully approved drug in our society. Its use is even encouraged by extensive advertising that makes smokers seem mature and sexually appealing. Our government actively supports the tobacco industry with public funds. Certainly, this is an example of how our division of drugs into good and evil is not at all rational.

New World Indians used tobacco in religious and magical rituals thousands of years ago, and some South American Indians still use strong tobacco as a consciousness-altering drug today. On special occasions they build giant cigars that the men take turns inhaling. They quickly become very intoxicated. Because they do not use tobacco except on special occasions, they have no tolerance to its effects and so get very high. When the Spanish discovered America, they observed Indians using tobacco and began using it themselves.

In the 1500s, Europeans also used tobacco to alter consciousness. It was a scarce and precious substance from the New World, and people smoked it occasionally, inhaling as deeply as they could and holding the smoke in their lungs to maximize the effect. Early tobacco was so harsh that people could not do this often enough to develop rapid tolerance and addiction. Still, authorities at the time were very upset at what they considered to be a new form of evil and tried their best to prohibit tobacco use. In many countries the penalty for people caught possessing tobacco was death.

Needless to say, these measures did not work, as criminal penalties for drug use never do. More and more people began smoking more and more regularly. As tobacco became increasingly common, it lost its special significance, and its users, instead of getting high on it once in a while, became addicts who needed it just to feel normal. The development of milder tobaccos that could be inhaled deeply and often gave birth to cigarette addiction as we know it today and with it the rise of the modern tobacco industry. Authorities then came to accept tobacco, eventually even encouraging its use in the belief that it promoted concentration and relaxation.

A recent British government study of adolescents shows that a youngster who smokes more than *one* cigarette has only a

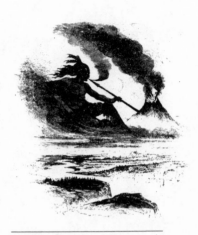

The Great Spirit of Native American religion, pictured as a cosmic pipe smoker. (Fitz Hugh Ludlow Memorial Library)

15 percent chance of remaining a nonsmoker. If you are thinking about experimenting with tobacco, especially in the form of cigarettes, consider the fact that most experimenters fall into this trap and become addicts before they know it.

Four Exotic Stimulant Plants

Betel.   Betel nut is the seed of a tropical palm tree with a spicy taste. In Asia, millions of people chew it daily, combining it with a pinch of lime (the alkaline mineral, not the fruit) and wrapping it in a fresh leaf of another plant called the betel pepper. This combination produces a great deal of red juice, which betel chewers spit out. The juice stains their teeth black over time. Betel nut contains a drug called arecoline, a stimulant comparable to caffeine. Betel chewing is a habit that is similar to the habits of chewing gum and drinking coffee or cola drinks in industrialized societies.

Qat (khat, chat, miraa).   Qat is a popular stimulant in a wide area of East Africa and the Middle East. It is a shrubby tree, whose fresh leaves and young twigs are eaten for their stimulating effect. The leaves lose their power when they dry out. Qat contains many active chemicals, some of which resemble amphetamines in their structure. Unlike coca, the leaves of qat, which have a bitter, astringent taste, are usually swallowed. Truck drivers in Kenya are big users of this plant.

Harvesting betel nuts. (Courtesy of the Swiss Federal Institute of Technology)

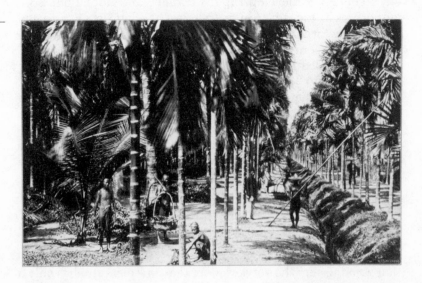

Yohimbe.   Yohimbe, the bark of an African tree with a bitter, spicy taste, contains a drug called yohimbine that is used in a few prescription medicines. Yohimbe bark is available at some herb stores and can be brewed into a stimulating tea. It is supposed to be an aphrodisiac, and some users say it causes tingling feelings along the spine.

Ephedra.   Ephedras are leafless bushes that grow in deserts throughout the world. They are related to pine trees and bear tiny cones. Several species contain the drug ephedrine, a stimulant and a remedy for asthma. American ephedra, found throughout the western United States, is known as Mormon tea because early Mormon settlers used it instead of caffeine beverages, which are prohibited by their religion. Herb stores sell both American ephedra and the stronger, Chinese type. The dry stems are boiled with water to make a pleasant-tasting tea that can be very stimulating.

Over-the-Counter (OTC) Drugs
Many cold remedies and other over-the-counter preparations contain caffeine to offset the drowsiness caused by antihistamines.* Another nonprescription stimulant in these products is the synthetic drug phenylpropanolamine. Recently it has appeared in over-the-counter diet pills with names such as Dexatrim. These sound like brand names of amphetamines. Like all stimulants, they may decrease appetite temporarily, but if used regularly for a long time, they make people dependent more often than thin.

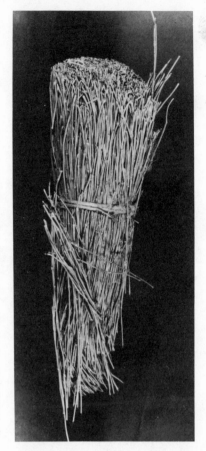

Dried Chinese ephedra.
(Dody Fugate)

Some Rules for Using Stimulants Safely

Because stimulants are so common, most people will use one or another at some time. If you become involved with stimulants, here are some rules that will help you stay in a good relationship with them.
1. *Limit your frequency of use.* All trouble with stimulants arises from using them too often. If you like the feeling a stimulant gives, it is all too easy to let your frequency of use creep up. Set limits! For example, never take a stimulant two days in a row.

*See pages 145–46 for a description of the effects of antihistamines.

2. *Use stimulants purposefully.* Taking these drugs just to feel good will not help you limit your use. If you are going to take a stimulant, you should use the stimulation for something — a physical or mental task, for instance. One side benefit of such purposeful use is that the satisfaction of accomplishment will offset the letdown when the drug wears off.

3. *Do not take stimulants to help you perform ordinary functions.* You should be able to get up in the morning, move your bowels, and make it through the afternoon without drugs. If you cannot, you should change your patterns of diet, sleep, and exercise. Relying on stimulants for everyday activity leads to too-frequent use and dependence.

4. *Take stimulants by mouth.* Putting these drugs more directly into the bloodstream (as by snorting, smoking, or shooting) accentuates the letdown following the up and encourages frequent administration. It also increases the harmful effects on the body.

5. *Take dilute forms of stimulants rather than concentrated ones.* The more dilute the preparation of a stimulant, the easier it is for the body to adjust to it, and the more gentle the letdown at the end. Preparations of plants such as coffee and tea are naturally more dilute than refined or synthetic drugs, and are easier to stay in good relationships with.

6. *Maintain good habits of nutrition, rest, and exercise.* Remember that stimulants force your body to give up its stores of chemical energy. Whenever you use stimulants, especially if you take them with any regularity, it is important to let your body recharge itself. The healthier you are, the less you will feel you need outside stimulation.

7. *Do not combine stimulants with depressants or other drugs.* Combinations of drugs always complicate matters. Some people can't sleep at night because they take too many stimulants during the day. So they take depressants at night. Then they can't get moving in the morning and have to take more stimulants. This pattern of drug-taking quickly leads to trouble.

8. *Avoid look-alike drugs.* They have nothing to recommend them.

It should not be difficult to use stimulants wisely and stay in good relationships with them. They are not answers to the ups and downs of life, and taking them to try to avoid the downs only leads to problems. Nor do they give anything for nothing.

Users pay later for any energy and good feeling stimulants give them. If you remain aware of what stimulants are and how they work, you will be able to avoid the trap of becoming dependent on them.

Suggested Reading

Some good information on the caffeine-containing plants will be found in Robert S. de Ropp's *Drugs and the Mind* (New York: Grove Press, 1960), an older book that is still one of the best and most readable references on psychoactive drugs. Coffee and tea are the subjects of *The Book of Coffee and Tea* by Meri Shardin (New York: St. Martin's Press, 1975). The most famous work on tea is Kakuzo Okakura's *The Book of Tea* (New York: Dover, 1964), first published in 1906. It is about much more than tea, being an elegant treatise on Japanese culture and philosophy written to help dispel Western misconceptions about Japan. A recent work on the same subject is *Tea: The Eyelids of Bodhidharma* by Eelco Hesse (Berkeley, California: And/Or Press, 1982). An interesting book on the origins and development of Coca-Cola is *The Big Drink: The Story of Coca-Cola* by E. J. Kahn, Jr. (New York: Random House, 1960). Chocolate devotees may be interested in a recently published book called *Chocolate: The Consuming Passion* by Sandra Boynton (New York: Workman, 1982), a profile and ardent defense of that substance by a self-proclaimed chocoholic.

W. Golden Mortimer's *History of Coca: Divine Plant of the Incas* (Berkeley, California: And/Or Press, 1974) was first published in 1901. It is a long description of Incan civilization, Peru, and coca and contains valuable information. A good excerpt from it is combined with writings of other authors in *The Coca Leaf and Cocaine Papers*, edited by George Andrews and David Solomon (New York: Harcourt Brace Jovanovich, 1975). *Mama Coca* by Antonil (London: Hassle Free Press, 1978) is a modern account of use of the leaf by Indians in Colombia that discusses the political aspects of coca.

Richard Ashley's *Cocaine: Its History, Uses, and Effects* (New York: St. Martin's Press, 1975) is a report on cocaine in Europe and America, from the time of its isolation from coca leaf in the late 1800s to the present. A more technical book and general reference on the subject is *Cocaine: A Drug and Its Social Evolution* by Lester Grinspoon and James B. Bakalar (New York: Basic Books, 1976). *The Seven Per Cent Solution* by

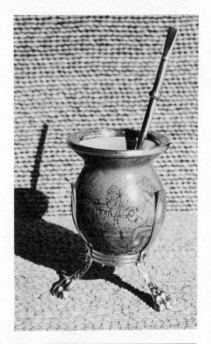

Argentinians drink maté — their national caffeine-containing drink — from decorated gourds. *Maté* means "gourd" in Spanish. (Woodward A. Wickham)

Nicholas Meyer (New York: Dutton, 1974) is a novel that concerns Sherlock Holmes's cocaine habit. It was made into a popular movie. The problems and perils of freebasing cocaine are brilliantly depicted by comedian Richard Pryor in his movie *Richard Pryor Live on the Sunset Strip.* Pryor's real-life habit of freebasing cocaine resulted in a near-fatal accident.

Despite widespread use, amphetamines have attracted less attention from writers than cocaine. One of the few books on the subject is *The Speed Culture: Amphetamine Use and Abuse in America* by Lester Grinspoon and Peter Hedblom (Cambridge, Massachusetts: Harvard University Press, 1975). It is technical in spots and not light reading. Arnold J. Mandell's *The Nightmare Season* (New York: Random House, 1976) is a doctor's account of problems of professional football players, in which amphetamines figure prominently. *The Tranquilizing of America: Pill Popping and the American Way of Life* by Richard Hughes and Robert Brewin (New York: Harcourt Brace Jovanovich, 1979) discusses medical uses of amphetamines, especially to control hyperactive children.

The lack of good books about tobacco is even more striking, considering that drug's popularity. *The Book of Pipes and Tobacco* by Carl Ehwa, Jr. (New York: Random House, 1974), gives general information. *To Smoke or Not To Smoke* by Luthor L. Terry and Daniel Horn (New York: Lothrop, Lee & Shepard, 1969) looks at reasons why people start smoking and also gives a history of tobacco. John Barth's novel *The Sot-Weed Factor* (New York: Bantam Books, 1969) revolves around tobacco. Probably the best account of cigarette addiction occurs in a comic novel by Italo Svevo, *Further Confessions of Zeno* (Berkeley: University of California Press, 1969). The author describes the endless tricks and self-deceptions used by a hooked smoker, as well as the low probability of cure.

7

Depressants

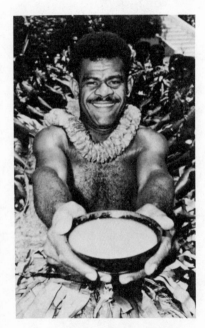

In a kava ceremony on the island of Fiji, a leader of the ritual offers a bowl of the prepared drink to arriving guests. Kava is a natural depressant.

DEPRESSANTS ARE DRUGS that lower the energy level of the nervous system, reducing sensitivity to outside stimulation and, in high doses, inducing sleep. Many depressants are used medically and socially and many are consumed illegally. In fact, depressants include some of the most popular drugs affecting mood.

At first glance, it may seem odd that people would want to take substances in order to depress their nervous systems. Who wants to feel groggy and depressed? Actually, depressants make people sleepy and stuporous only in high doses; in lower doses they often make people relaxed and happy. Alcohol is a good example. One or two drinks can make people feel cheerful, alert, and more alive, while three or four can make them drunk, with obvious symptoms of reduced brain function.

Scientists don't really know why low doses of depressants make people feel stimulated. One theory is that the first parts of the brain to be depressed are inhibitory centers that normally act to dampen mood. As the dose is increased, more and more parts of the nervous system are slowed down. Very high doses of depressants can cause coma, in which all consciousness is lost; a person in a coma is insensible to all input — even loud noise and intense pain. Still higher doses of these drugs can shut down the most vital centers in the brain, such as the one that controls respiration, resulting in a quick death from lack of oxygen.

Depressant drugs are more dangerous than stimulants because overdoses of them are apt to kill people by interfering with vital brain centers. Also, they produce a wider variety of effects, from relaxation and euphoria in low doses to unresponsive coma in very high doses.

Depressants include several distinct categories of drugs, each with its own benefits and dangers.

Sedative-Hypnotics

This large category of depressants comprises alcohol, "sleeping pills," and certain tranquilizers. In low doses these drugs promote relaxation and restfulness (sedation), especially in the daytime. Larger doses, especially at night, induce sleep (the word *hypnosis* comes from the name of the Greek god of sleep). "Sedative-hypnotic" refers to this double action.

Alcohol (Ethyl Alcohol, Ethanol)

Alcohol is the most popular psychoactive drug in the world, used every day by many millions of people. Probably, it is also the oldest drug known to human beings, because it is easy to discover that fruits and juices, left to stand in a warm place, soon ferment into alcoholic mixtures. Alcohol is so commonplace and its effects, both good and bad, are so well known that they need little description. Anyone who has felt the pleasant stimulation of a glass of wine knows the beneficial side of this drug. Anyone who has interacted with a drunk person knows how powerful and unpleasant alcohol can be in overdose. Anyone who has lived with an alcoholic can attest to the horrors of alcohol addiction.

Production of ethyl alcohol depends upon yeast, which feeds on sugar, making alcohol and carbon dioxide as by-products. Yeasts are simple, one-celled forms of life found everywhere — in the air and on the skins of many fruits, especially grapes. To grow and multiply, yeast cells need water, sugar, and warmth. They keep on growing until they use up all the sugar or until the rising concentration of alcohol kills them. Alcohol is a poison as well as a drug; in high enough doses it kills living things, including the yeasts that make it.

Natural sources of sugar available to primitive people were fruit and honey, both of which can be made into wine with a maximum alcohol content of about 12 percent. Starch is also a potential source of alcohol, but it must be converted to sugar by

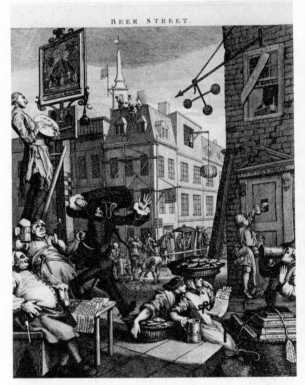

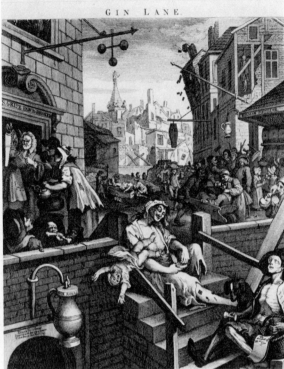

enzymes before yeast can digest it. There are enzymes in saliva that can accomplish this, and one of the earliest kinds of beer was made by Indians in tropical America who learned to chew corn to a pulp, spit it into clay pots, mix it with water, and let it ferment. Sprouting grains also produce usable enzymes; in standard beer-making, sprouted barley (malt) is used to convert the starch of grains to sugar so that yeast can grow and produce alcohol. The alcohol content of beer is usually less than half that of wine. Beer is also more nutritious than wine because it has a lot of calories in the form of carbohydrates.

Distilled alcohol is a relatively new product, dating back only a few hundred years. Brandy was the first distilled liquor made; it was obtained by heating wine and then cooling and condensing the vapors in another container. This process increases the alcohol content dramatically: from 12 percent up to 40 or 50 percent. The original idea of distillers was to concentrate wine to a smaller volume to make it easier to ship it in barrels overseas. At the end of the voyage the brandy was to be diluted with water back to an alcohol content of 12 percent.

In these famous drawings the English artist William Hogarth (1697–1764) portrayed the different consequences of regular use of fermented and distilled alcoholic beverages. The residents of Beer Street are happy, healthy, and productive, maintaining an orderly neighborhood. In Gin Lane there is disorder, chaos, and death. Among other calamities: a man has hanged himself, a skeletal man is near death from malnutrition, and a drunken woman lets her helpless child fall to its doom. (The Boston Athenaeum)

What happened, of course, was that when people got their hands on what was in the barrels, no one waited to add water. Suddenly a new and powerful form of alcohol flooded the world.

Our society now manufactures and consumes many distilled liquors. Scotch and bourbon whiskeys are made from beerlike preparations of grain. Rum is distilled from fermented molasses; gin and vodka are just diluted ethyl alcohol (gin has flavor added), also usually distilled from grain. Because of their much higher alcohol content, these hard liquors are stronger and more intoxicating than fermented drinks.

From earliest times, people probably used beer and wine much as we use them today: as social and recreational drugs, to dispel worry and anxiety, to feel high, and as a change from the dull routines of work. Our early ancestors probably also noticed that the effects of alcohol were variable and dose-related, and that some people became dependent on it.

Alcohol is absorbed very quickly from the digestive system, enters the bloodstream, and reaches the brain, where it causes its effects on mood and behavior. The body has to work hard to eliminate alcohol; it burns some of it as fuel and excretes some unchanged in the breath and urine. The burden of metabolizing alcohol falls especially on the liver.

The effects of alcohol are directly related to how much of it is in the blood at any time. Low concentrations, particularly at the beginning of drinking, cause alertness, good moods, feelings of energy, warmth, and confidence, and the dissipation of anxiety and inhibition. Most people find these changes pleasant.

It is important to note, however, that some of the sensations — especially the sense of confidence — produced by low doses of alcohol may be false. Unlike stimulants, alcohol and other depressants slow the functioning of the nervous system, including reflexes, reaction time, and efficiency of muscular response. Though people often feel they are performing better after a few drinks, scientific tests show otherwise. This is one source of danger in using depressant drugs to feel good: the false sense of confidence can lead people to take unwarranted risks, such as driving cars in conditions that favor disaster.

Similarly, the sense of warmth produced by drinking is deceptive. It is due to increased blood flow to the skin, which allows more heat to radiate to the outside of the body. In fact, inner body temperature is dropping even as the sensation of warmth increases, so that people inadequately dressed for cold weather who drink in order to feel warm may fall victim to hypothermia.

I like alcohol. It is a powerful drug and, God knows, for some people a hellish one, but if used carefully it can give great pleasure. After a long, hard day, the splendid warm glow that strong drink provides is one of my favorite feelings; it starts in the pit of my stomach, then spreads to my limbs and brain. I know that alcohol is a depressant, but it acts and feels like a gentle relaxant — of the spirit as well as of the physical body. Just notice the increased vivacity and noise level at a cocktail party after a drink has been served to see how alcohol can put people at ease emotionally. — sixty-two-year-old man, psychoanalyst

Another example of the deceptive nature of alcohol is its sexual effect. Many people who drink to enhance sex claim that alcohol increases desire, removes inhibitions, and promotes relaxation. In men, however, its depression of the nervous system can prevent erection and drastically interfere with sexual performance. Writers as far back as Shakespeare have noted this property of alcohol. In Act II, Scene 3, of *Macbeth*, the following exchange occurs between Macduff and a porter in Macbeth's castle:

MACDUFF: What three things does drink especially provoke?
PORTER: Marry, sir, nose painting, sleep, and urine. Lechery, sir, it provokes, and unprovokes; it provokes the desire, but it takes away the performance.

People who drink should be aware that their subjective impressions while under the influence of alcohol may not correspond to reality.

Further, it is clear that, as with any psychoactive drug, the pleasant feelings alcohol can provide depend as much on set and setting as on pharmacological action. The same amount of wine that makes someone pleasantly high at a party may make a depressed person in a lonely room even more depressed.

Concentration of alcohol in the bloodstream is determined by several factors: first, by the concentration of alcohol in the drink; second, by the rate of drinking; third, by the presence or absence of food in the stomach; and fourth, by the rate at which the body can metabolize and eliminate alcohol.

The stronger the drink, the faster the blood alcohol level will rise and the sooner a person will get drunk. Gulping down cocktails and drinking wine like water are good ways to speed through the more pleasant, early effects of alcohol intoxication and go right to the less desirable ones.

Food in the stomach, especially milk, slows down absorption of alcohol into the blood. Therefore, drinking on an empty stomach can result in faster and more intense drunkenness. Eating before and during drinking moderates the intensity of alcohol's effects.

Finally, some people metabolize alcohol more rapidly than others and so can handle larger doses. People who drink alcohol regularly metabolize it faster than people who do not, and won't be affected by doses that nondrinkers would certainly feel. This is tolerance, and it develops quickly to alcohol and other sedative-hypnotics. Alcoholics show very high tolerance to the drug;

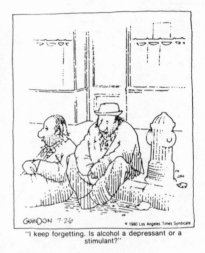

"I keep forgetting. Is alcohol a depressant or a stimulant?"

(Copyright © 1980 *Los Angeles Times* Syndicate. Reprinted with permission)

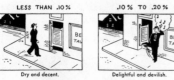

DEGREES OF INTOXICATION

The percentages indicated show the concentration of alcohol in the blood, brain, and other organs.

The cartoons here used are adapted from a paper by Emil Bogen.

From *Effects of Alcoholic Drinks, Tobacco, Sedatives, Narcotics* by Thurman B. Rice, M.D., and Rolla N. Harger, Ph.D. (Chicago: Wheeler Publishing Co., 1952)

they can even survive doses of alcohol that would kill nondrinkers. Other people may have lower than normal abilities to metabolize alcohol. Some Japanese, for example, have an inborn biochemical quirk that causes them to get drunk on doses of wine or liquor that would hardly affect most Americans or Europeans.

As alcohol increases in the bloodstream, it depresses more and more of the nervous system, producing the familiar symptoms of drunkenness: slurred speech, incoordination, insensitivity to pain, and inappropriate behavior. People become drunk in very different ways, depending on their personalities, their mood at the time, and the social setting. Some people become boisterous and obnoxious; others become overly friendly, confiding the most intimate details of their lives to perfect strangers. Some people get belligerent, even violent, while others become gloomy, tearful, and self-pitying.

Drunkenness is a serious problem throughout the world, accounting for many accidents, acts of violence, injuries, and deaths. Many traffic accidents are directly related to alcohol intoxication, as are many murders. It isn't uncommon for drunk people to kill friends or relatives and have no memory of the incidents the next day, a consequence of alcohol's depressant effect on parts of the brain responsible for reason, thought, and memory.

Most people who get drunk eventually fall into stuporous sleep. When they wake up they are hung over, with such symptoms as sour stomach, headache, weakness, shakiness, depression, and inability to concentrate, work, or think clearly. These symptoms reflect the toxic effects of alcohol on the body and are very uncomfortable. Alcohol is strongly diuretic — that is, it increases the flow of urine, causing the body to lose water. A night of hard drinking can result in serious dehydration if lost water is not replaced, and this condition may contribute to the discomfort of the next day's hangover.

Because additional alcohol ("the hair of the dog that bit you") makes a hung-over person feel better in the short run, excessive drinking can lead to further drinking and start people on the path to dependence.

Dependence on alcohol is a true addiction, marked by extreme craving for the drug, tolerance, and withdrawal. The craving for alcohol among alcoholics is legendary and has been the subject of many books and films.* Recovered alcoholics tell frightening stories of the lengths to which they went to obtain

*See page 90.

WINGTIPS

by Michael Goodman

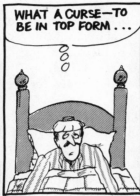

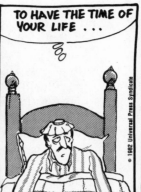

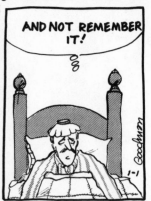

their drug when deprived, and of squandering all of their money and that of their families on drink. Withdrawal from alcohol is a major medical crisis. Some of its worst forms, such as delirium tremens (the D.T.'s), can be fatal and are more serious than withdrawal from narcotics.

Moreover, because alcohol is such a strong and toxic drug, prolonged regular use can cause tremendous physical damage. Cirrhosis of the liver, in which normal liver cells are replaced by useless fibrous tissue, is a direct and common result of overuse of alcohol and leads to many distressing symptoms, among them loss of sexual potency and inability to digest food. The other organs that bear the brunt of alcohol's poisonous effect are the brain and nervous system. Alcoholics develop shakes, amnesia, and loss of intellect, which may reflect permanent damage to nerves. The list of medical problems associated with excessive drinking is much too long to reproduce here. It includes adverse effects on unborn babies of alcoholic mothers and increased susceptibility to such infectious diseases as pneumonia and tuberculosis. Hospitals around the world are filled with chronic medical patients whose bodies are ravaged by alcohol.

Alcoholism is also one of the most stubborn forms of drug addiction, very resistant to treatment. Many doctors who work with alcoholics admit they have little success with them. The only groups that seem to be able to help are Alcoholics Anonymous, which depends on an almost religious adherence to a group ethic, and the Native American Church, which uses peyote in religious rituals and vigorously crusades against drinking among American Indians.*

*See pages 105–6.

Not all regular drinkers become alcoholics. In fact, most regular drinkers are not addicted. Possibly, some people are prone to become addicts because of peculiarities of their biochemistry or metabolism. Children of alcoholics are more likely to grow up to be alcoholics, but so are children of families where both parents are teetotalers. That suggests that the lack in childhood of good role models for healthy drinking may be an important factor.

One of the clearest signs of alcoholism is repeated drinking to get drunk. Alcoholics cannot limit their intake to a social drink or two; they invariably go much further. But drunkenness isn't much fun, either at the time or the following day. Why, then, do so many people consume overdoses of alcohol?

This question points up the main problem with alcohol. As noted earlier, most people like the early effects of the drug, which resemble those of stimulants, but taking more of it dramatically changes the quality of the effects. It isn't easy for people to learn how to stay within the dose range that makes them feel good; it is very easy to cross into the zone of unpleasant effects and regret it. Young people beginning to drink should recognize that this is a problem they will have to deal with by acquiring experience. Many people — if they are metabolically normal, come from supportive families, and don't have serious psychological problems — learn how to control their intake of alcohol and keep from sliding into the trouble zone, but others do not.

Alcohol is one of the most difficult drugs to control because it is so strong and because the dose-related difference in its effects is so great. Used intelligently, alcohol can be useful in relieving stress. Some people even claim that alcohol promotes health. For example, some medical studies suggest that moderate drinking decreases the risk of heart attacks in later life. Wine lovers say that drinking wine with meals aids digestion. Some physicians think old people benefit from alcohol in small amounts. These claims may be true. Unfortunately, some people cannot learn to drink moderately. Recovered alcoholics, for example, usually become drunks again very quickly if they try to drink socially.

There is no question that alcohol is the most toxic of all the drugs discussed in this book. Yet our own society has made alcohol its social drug of choice. It is widely available in many attractive forms, extensively advertised, and used to the point that it is hard to avoid. In certain groups liquor is so much the required social lubricant that nondrinkers feel uncomfortable

Although I kept trying to use alcohol moderately, whenever I'd set out to get high on it, I would always keep on drinking till I got drunk, no matter how many resolutions I made not to . . . I've tried various drugs since those days and don't think anything comes close to alcohol in terms of raw strength and potential for trouble. I couldn't learn to control it well, and I see many people around me who have the same problem.
— thirty-seven-year-old man, college professor

and out of place. Alcohol comes into people's lives at every turn. Friends give each other bottles of liquor as holiday gifts. Airlines sell drinks in flight and placate passengers with free drinks if planes are subject to undue delays. On billboards and in magazines the pleasures of drinking are everywhere extolled. Everyone in our society must learn to come to terms with this powerful drug.

Unless you are a Muslim or a Mormon or belong to some other group that prohibits its use altogether, you will have to learn how to refuse alcohol if you don't want to drink or how to drink it intelligently and not let your use get out of control.

Some Suggestions for Using Alcohol Wisely

1. Define what benefits you want from alcohol. Remember that alcohol is attractive because it can make people feel temporarily better, both physically and mentally. You can enjoy these good effects if you learn to use the drug carefully and purposefully. If you feel feverish and achy from flu, going to bed and taking a small drink may be a good remedy. If you walk into a party and feel awkward, anxious, and inhibited, a little alcohol may help you get into the swing of things.

2. It is good to make rules about when and where *not* to drink. For example, a person who uses alcohol to relax after a hard day shouldn't drink at the end of an easy one, or before a day is done. No one should drink and drive.

3. Rules about times, places, and situations that are appropriate for drinking help control the tendency of alcohol to get out of hand. People might decide they will drink with friends but not by themselves, on weekends and holidays but not during the week, after sunset but not during the day.

4. Learn to regulate the amount of alcohol in your bloodstream. Once it's there, only time can get it out. You can control the rate of absorption of alcohol into your blood by drinking dilute forms of it rather than concentrated ones (for example, by adding water to wine and mixers to hard liquor). You can also make sure you have food in your stomach before and during drinking. You can practice consuming alcoholic drinks slowly. Finally, you can practice saying no to further drinks when you've had enough.

5. Whenever you consume alcohol heavily, remember to

drink plenty of plain water to offset fluid losses from increased urination. By doing so you may moderate the next day's hangover.

6. Don't spend time with people who drink to excess or encourage you to drink more than you want.

7. Be careful about falling into patterns of regular drinking to deal with ongoing emotional problems, such as anxiety or depression. Alcohol may mask the symptoms temporarily, but it cannot solve the problems, and this kind of use is more likely to lead to dependence.

8. Adolescence, with its confusions, peer pressures, and tendencies to rebel, is a time when unhealthy patterns of drug use can develop that may persist into later life and be very hard to break. Young people may think they aren't as susceptible to dependence on alcohol as adults, but the evidence contradicts this view. Alcohol is a difficult drug to control at any age, and alcoholism doesn't appear overnight. It is the result of unwise drinking over time, beginning with the earliest experience of the drug.

9. Alcohol contains calories. If you are trying to lose weight, watch your intake.

10. If you drink regularly, make sure you maintain good habits of rest, exercise, and nutrition.

11. If you begin to suspect you have problems with drinking, or if people who know you think you do, seek help from professionals. It is difficult or impossible to deal with problem drinking without outside help.

The manufacturer of this strong liqueur seems to be recommending solitary drinking, a practice that favors abuse and can be a sign of alcoholism.

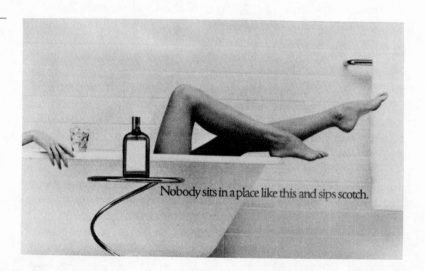

Nobody sits in a place like this and sips scotch.

Barbiturates and Other Sleeping Pills ("Downers")

This class of sedative-hypnotic drugs — loosely known as sleeping pills, or downers — has been around for some time. They are manufactured both legally and illegally, and are widely used. Medical doctors prescribe these substances in low doses to calm people during the day and in higher doses to help them sleep at night. There are millions of people who take sleeping pills every night and think they can't fall asleep without them. Millions of others take downers for nonmedical reasons: to get high, to feel good, or to party.

Barbituric acid was discovered in 1864. Since then a number of derivatives of it have been introduced. They are all known as barbiturates and are the most important drugs in this class. The first barbiturate sleeping drug, called barbital, appeared in 1903. The second, called phenobarbital, appeared in 1912. Hundreds of barbiturates are now known, and many are currently in use.

Some of the barbiturates are slowly metabolized and eliminated by the kidneys. Barbital and phenobarbital are in this group, and are known as long-acting barbiturates because their effects last twelve to twenty-four hours. They are used as daytime sedatives more than as nighttime hypnotics, and since they don't produce much euphoria or stimulation, few people take them to get high.

Another group of barbiturates is more rapidly metabolized by the liver. Their effects last six or seven hours, and they are called short-acting. They include amobarbital (Amytal), pentobarbital (Nembutal), hexobarbital (Sombulex), and secobarbital (Seconal). These drugs behave very much like alcohol, giving pleasant feelings in low doses, especially as they begin to take effect. Therefore, some people seek them out to change the way they feel, and there is no shortage of them on the black market.

Finally, there are very short-acting barbiturates that produce almost immediate unconsciousness when injected intravenously. Thiopental (Pentothal) is the main example; dentists and doctors use it as an anesthetic for surgical operations. Since it wipes out awareness so fast and leaves no memory of the experience, no one takes it for fun.

When people talk about taking downers they usually mean the short-acting barbiturates or a few similar drugs that will be mentioned later. All of these substances are like alcohol, and most of the statements in the alcohol section apply to downers as well.* Sleeping pills can make people feel and look drunk, can

*See pages 60–68.

leave users with hangovers, can kill when taken in overdose by knocking out the respiratory center of the brain, and can produce stubborn addiction with dangerous withdrawal syndromes, marked, in some cases, by convulsions and death.

Since the similarities between downers and alcohol are so numerous, it might be easier to talk about how they differ.

Unlike alcohol, sleeping pills are noncaloric; the body cannot burn them as fuel but must metabolize them in other ways. They are also not as toxic as alcohol over time and don't cause the kind of liver disease and other medical damage so common in alcoholics. Tolerance to downers occurs, as with alcohol, but there is an important and curious difference. As people use them regularly, tolerance to the effects on mood develops faster than tolerance to the lethal dose. For this reason, people run a greater risk of accidentally killing themselves with these substances. For example, people who get into the habit of taking sleeping pills every night to fall asleep might start out with one a night, progress to two, then graduate to four to get the same effect. One night the dose they need to fall asleep might also be the dose that stops their breathing.

It is especially dangerous to combine alcohol and downers because their depressant effects are additive. A dose of alcohol a person is used to plus a dose of a downer that would be all right by itself may add up to coma and death. Many people have died because they were ignorant of this fact.

As with alcohol, the effects of downers on mood are extremely variable, depending on individual personality, expectation, and setting. Some people who take sleeping pills feel nothing but sleepiness. Others fight off the sleepiness and say they feel high. A dose of Seconal taken at a wild party might inspire violent excitement, whereas a person taking the same dose in a quiet room might be overcome with lethargy. Some medical patients have strange reactions to prescribed downers, becoming anxious and agitated instead of calmed down. Old people are likely to become intoxicated on ordinary doses, as are people with liver or kidney disease.

Most people take these drugs by mouth, but injectable forms are available. In hospitals, hypnotic doses of Nembutal are often given by intramuscular injection, especially to patients who cannot take medicine by mouth. On the street, some users inject barbiturates intravenously (sometimes crushing and dissolving oral preparations), a practice that greatly increases their toxicity.

Other users like to combine downers and stimulants, claiming that the combined effect is more pleasant. A few such com-

The barbiturate addict presents a shocking spectacle. He cannot coordinate, he staggers, falls off bar stools, goes to sleep in the middle of a sentence, drops food out of his mouth. He is confused, quarrelsome, and stupid. And he almost always uses other drugs, anything he can lay his hands on: alcohol, benzedrine, opiates, marijuana. Barbiturate users are looked down on in addict society: "Goof ball bums. They got no class to them." . . . It seems to me that barbiturates cause the worst possible form of addiction, unsightly, deteriorating, difficult to treat.
— *William S. Burroughs, from his novel* Naked Lunch *(1959)*

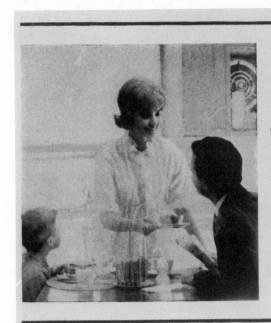

That "good morning" feeling... thanks to

*

glutethimide

The morning feeling after taking a sedative is more likely to be a hangover than what is pictured here.

binations are even legally made for medical use. One example, Dexamyl, is a mixture of amobarbital and dextroamphetamine (Dexedrine). Supposedly, the barbiturate counteracts any tendency of the amphetamine to cause anxiety or jitteriness, while the amphetamine reinforces the potential of the barbiturate to produce euphoria. Similarly, people who use a lot of cocaine say that drinking alcohol at the same time reduces the unpleasant side effects of that drug, while the cocaine keeps them from getting drunk and minimizes hangovers. Although these combinations probably do no harm when used occasionally, they may have a higher potential for abuse in the long run because they make it easier to take larger quantities of drugs.

Dependence on barbiturates can occur in both medical patients and street users. Doctors write vast numbers of prescriptions for sleeping pills, and many people fall into the habit of taking them every night. Certainly, it is appropriate to take these drugs when insomnia is temporary and due to a specific, identifiable cause. For instance, the death of a close friend or relative, the breakup of a family, the loss of a job, even moving, may produce serious disturbances of sleep, and sleeping pills may help during the crisis. Some people take these drugs to help them sleep on long plane flights, during other kinds of travel, after periods of intense work or stress, and when working shifts.

There is no question that Quaalude can be dangerous when used irresponsibly, or that it can be addicting. As a recreational drug, taken on occasion in a responsible manner, it seems to me safe and interesting and gives me an experience different from anything else.
— thirty-six-year-old man, drug counselor

There is no harm in taking sleeping pills a few nights in a row in such situations.

Problems arise when people take them every night over a long time. Persistent insomnia is always a symptom of other trouble, either physical or emotional. Sleeping pills treat the symptom only. Moreover, the sleep induced by downers is not the same as natural sleep. It doesn't provide as much dreaming time, for one thing, and is likely to be followed by a slight hangover. Because drug-induced sleep may not supply all the needs of body and mind, it may, over time, aggravate an underlying problem. Although many people take sleeping pills regularly for years without having to increase the dose or suffering any obvious difficulties, this kind of usage is a form of drug dependence.

Taking downers as a means of dealing with feelings of depression or low self-esteem is probably the riskiest way of using them. Like alcohol, these drugs may mask the symptoms temporarily, but over time they often increase anxiety and depression, encouraging further drug-taking in a downward spiral that can end in suicide.

As noted earlier, there are a number of nonbarbiturate downers, the most popular of which is methaqualone, marketed under such brand names as Quaalude, Sopor, and Mandrax. Its effects are equivalent to those of the barbiturates, although on its own it is less likely to depress the respiratory center in overdose. Still, deaths have occurred as a result of combinations of alcohol and methaqualone. Street users talk about "luding out" — that is, taking Quaaludes and wine to produce a numb, euphoric state. Quaalude has gained a street reputation as a sex enhancer and party drug. Like all downers, it can lower inhibitions and reduce anxiety in the same way as alcohol. But also like alcohol, it will interfere with sexual performance in males and may make it more difficult for women to experience orgasm. Fake Quaaludes — look-alike tablets containing no methaqualone — are commonly sold to gullible buyers on the black market.

Another downer, chloral hydrate, is the oldest sleeping drug still in medical use. Although rare today, abuse of it was not uncommon in the last century. Slipped into alcoholic drinks, it is the notorious "Mickey Finn" or "knockout drops" used to drug unsuspecting people into unconsciousness in order to rob or shanghai them.

Still other nonbarbiturate downers include glutethimide (Doriden), methyprylon (Noludar), ethchlorvynol (Placidyl), and paraldehyde. All of these drugs are used in medicine as hypnotics. They sometimes find their way to the black market, where users of illegal downers buy them. Their benefits and dangers are the same as those of the barbiturates.

Suggestions for Using Downers Safely

1. Take sleeping pills by mouth in doses no higher than those recommended by doctors, pharmacists, or manufacturers. (Often lower doses will do.)
2. Don't drive or operate machinery while under the influence of these drugs. Like alcohol, they impair judgment, coordination, and reflexes.
3. Exercise extreme caution about using downers in combination with alcohol or other depressant drugs.
4. Don't fall into the habit of relying on downers for sleep. Insomnia can usually be overcome by improving health; getting more exercise; cutting down on intake of stimulants, including caffeine and tobacco; taking warm baths before bed; and by many other means not involving drugs.
5. Be wary of relying on these drugs to get you out of bad moods.
6. Don't take downers regularly in combination with stimulants just because you like the feeling.
7. Don't take downers if you are ill, especially not if you have any liver or kidney problems, unless a doctor prescribes them for you.
8. If you find yourself becoming dependent on downers, with developing tolerance or any unusual physical or mental symptoms, seek professional help.

The Minor Tranquilizers

The third and last class of sedative-hypnotics consists of relatively new drugs, products of the modern pharmaceutical industry. Dating back only to the mid-1950s, these drugs are called minor tranquilizers, a misleading name. The word *minor* is supposed to distinguish them from the "major" tranquilizers — compounds such as chlorpromazine (Thorazine), which are used to manage psychotic patients.* Actually, these two kinds of tranquilizers are chemically and pharmacologically unrelated. Minor tranquilizers are not, as their name implies, mild drugs. There is nothing minor about their effects, the problems they can cause, or their potential for abuse.

Since their invention, the minor tranquilizers have achieved enormous popularity in medicine. Doctors have writ-

*See pages 141–43.

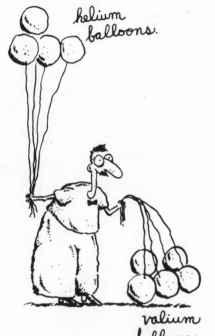

helium
balloons.

valium
balloons

ten millions upon millions of prescriptions for them, and pharmaceutical companies have made billions of dollars by promoting and selling them as antianxiety agents. In fact, more prescriptions are written for these compounds than for *any other drugs*.

The first minor tranquilizer to be released to the world was meprobamate; it appeared in 1954 under the brand name Miltown,* and within a short time after its appearance, people were holding Miltown parties — taking the drug socially and recreationally, just to get high.

The most popular minor tranquilizers appeared in the 1960s — a family of drugs called benzodiazepenes. Three of the most famous are chlordiazepoxide (Librium), diazepam (Valium), and flurazepam (Dalmane). The manufacturer of Librium and Valium, once a small company selling vitamins and antacids, is now one of the most powerful pharmaceutical corporations in the world.

The pharmaceutical industry has tried hard to convince doctors and patients that these chemicals are revolutionary drugs that specifically reduce anxiety, making people calm and relaxed. In fact, the minor tranquilizers are just another variation on the theme of alcohol and other sedative-hypnotics, with the same tendency to produce adverse effects and dependence.

Compared to barbiturates, the minor tranquilizers are safer in overdose, somewhat less dangerous in combination with alcohol, and not as likely to cause a dramatic withdrawal syndrome when long-term use is stopped. Also, the minor tranquilizers are useful in relaxing tense muscles. As daytime sedatives, they produce less drowsiness than barbiturates, but they can still make driving dangerous and interfere with other motor skills, as well as with clear thinking. As nighttime hypnotics, they induce sleep and may be preferable to barbiturates if anxiety or muscle tension is present or if patients need a sleeping pill for more than a few nights in a row.

Street users of the minor tranquilizers take them for the same reasons they take illegal downers: to improve mood, reduce anxiety and inhibitions, and promote social interaction.

In most cases, abuse of the minor tranquilizers, particularly of Valium, Librium, and Miltown, has resulted from irresponsible practices of marketing and prescribing. In promoting these drugs, the manufacturers portrayed stresses of everyday life as disease states treatable by prescribing their products. For ex-

*It was also marketed later as Equanil.

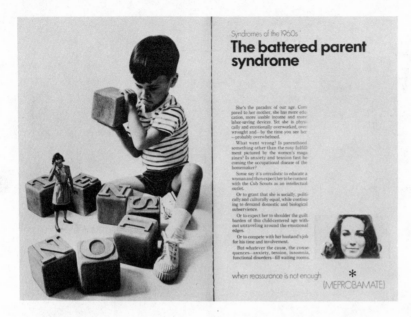

Syndromes of the 1960s
The battered parent syndrome

She's the paradox of our age. Compared to her mother, she has more education, more usable income and more labor-saving devices. Yet she is physically and emotionally overwrought, overwrought and—by the time you see her—probably overwhelmed.

What went wrong? Is parenthood something other than the rosy fulfillment pictured by the women's magazines? Is anxiety and tension fast becoming the occupational disease of the homemaker?

Some say it's unrealistic to educate a woman and then expect her to be content with the Cub Scouts as an intellectual outlet.

Or to grant that she is socially, politically and culturally equal, while continuing to demand domestic and biological subservience.

Or to expect her to shoulder the guilt burden of this child-centered age without unraveling around the emotional edges.

Or to compete with her husband's job for his time and involvement.

But whatever the cause, the consequences—anxiety, tension, insomnia, functional disorders—fill waiting rooms.

when reassurance is not enough *
(MEPROBAMATE)

ample, ads in medical journals recommended Librium for the college girl whose "newly stimulated intellectual curiosity may make her more sensitive to and apprehensive about unstable national and world conditions"; in other words, pop some Librium if the news freaks you out. Other ads have suggested giving tranquilizers to harried mothers and bored housewives, to "the woman who can't get along with her new daughter-in-law," and to "the newcomer in town who can't make friends."

Critics of this kind of salesmanship point out that women seem to be targets far more often than men. Just as pharmaceutical companies encouraged doctors to prescribe amphetamines to depressed housewives in the 1960s, they have since urged doctors to give Valium, Librium, and Miltown to anxious women. Increasing opposition to these practices has curtailed them to some extent.

Using tranquilizers to deal with everyday difficulties causes the same problem associated with all depressant drugs: long-term dependence. Even though the consequences of dependence on tranquilizers may be less severe than those of dependence on alcohol and barbiturates, the result is the same. There is no treatment of the underlying causes of anxiety, merely the creation of a legal drug habit.

The makers of Valium and Librium at one time pushed the idea of using these drugs to treat alcoholics, and many doctors

Pharmaceutical companies have sometimes invented new diseases to sell their products. Manufacturers of the minor tranquilizers were especially creative, as this example from the 1960s shows.

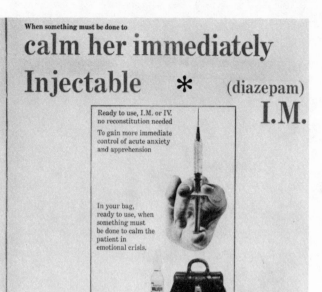

an Emotional Crisis...

Surgical emergencies often present you with a second patient as well, one with an acute emotional crisis: for example, the mother of the patient.

Emotionally distressed and upset, she may need your help almost as much as her child does.

When something must be done to

calm her immediately

Injectable * (diazepam)

I.M.

Ready to use, I.M. or IV. no reconstitution needed

To gain more immediate control of acute anxiety and apprehension

In your bag, ready to use, when something must be done to calm the patient in emotional crisis.

followed their advice. When the alcoholics drank less, the doctors imagined they had achieved something, but all they had really done was to substitute one sedative-hypnotic for another. (One expert on alcoholism has called Valium "whiskey in a pill.")

Throughout history, doctors have relied on mood-altering drugs to deal with difficult patients. Psychoactive drugs change the way people feel, satisfy patients' desires for medicine, and make doctors feel they have been useful — or at least make the patients go away. A hundred years ago, opium and alcohol were the mainstays of medical treatment along with cannabis (marijuana). At the turn of the century, cocaine was doled out for all sorts of complaints. Today, Librium and Valium are some of the most widely prescribed drugs in the world. Certainly, the minor tranquilizers have their place in medicine, but long-term use of them for people who are anxious, depressed, or unable to sleep is symptomatic treatment of the worst sort.

Suggestions for Avoiding Trouble with Tranquilizers

1. Be aware that these drugs are strong depressants, similar in effect to alcohol, and can cause unpleasant reactions and dependence.

2. All of the cautions about downers apply to the minor tranquilizers as well.
3. If you take these drugs, whether on medical prescription or for fun, don't use them every day. Take them intermittently or occasionally to avoid falling into a pattern of habitual use.

General Anesthetics

General anesthetics are powerful depressants used in surgery to make people insensible to pain. They are gases or volatile liquids administered by inhalation through masks over the face or tubes in the throat. Most are never seen outside operating rooms, but a few have been popular recreational drugs in the past, and one — nitrous oxide, or laughing gas — is still in common nonmedical use.

When breathed, general anesthetics enter the blood very rapidly, depressing brain function within seconds. The stronger ones quickly produce complete unconsciousness, a state that lasts as long as the drug is administered and for a short time afterward. Like all depressants, general anesthetics can kill by shutting down the respiratory center and other vital functions. During surgery, therefore, a specially trained doctor or technician must monitor the administration of the drugs and the moment-to-moment condition of the patient.

In low doses, general anesthetics produce changes in consciousness similar to alcohol and sedative-hypnotics, and for many years people have experimented with them to get high and to explore their minds.

Chloroform is one of the oldest drugs in this group. Since it is very toxic, it is no longer used. Years ago, people sometimes sniffed the fumes of liquid chloroform or swallowed small amounts in order to experience what disapproving critics called a "cheap drunk."

The era of surgical anesthesia began in 1846, when a dentist in Boston demonstrated that ether could safely render patients insensible to the pain of operations. Today ether (or, more correctly, diethyl ether) is still widely used to induce unconsciousness before surgery. Ether is a volatile liquid, easily administered to people through breathing masks. It has a strong chemical smell, and its main disadvantage is that its fumes make an extremely explosive mixture with air. Great care must be taken when ether is in use to prevent violent explosions from

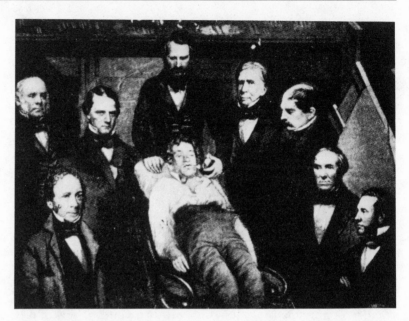

The first public demonstration of anesthesia; the anesthetic used was ether. Massachusetts General Hospital, 1846. (Courtesy of Massachusetts General Hospital, Boston)

WONDERFUL EFFECTS OF ETHER IN A CASE OF SCOLDING WIFE.

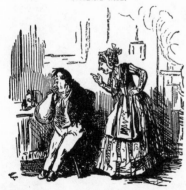

Patient.—" THIS IS REALLY QUITE DELIGHTFUL—A MOST BEAUTIFUL DREAM."

An English reaction to the discovery of ether (From *Punch*, 1847)

(Reproduced by permission of *Punch*)

accidental sparks or flames. Another disadvantage of ether is that overdoses of it rapidly put people into deep comas and stop their respiration.

Prior to 1846, surgery was horribly painful; patients had to be tied down, and their screams could be heard far from operating rooms. The discovery of ether anesthesia revolutionized surgery. Even before this event — as long ago as 1800 — ether was a well-known curiosity; many people played with it just to experience its unusual effects on consciousness.

Ether parties were popular throughout the 1800s. People would gather for the express purpose of sniffing the fumes or drinking tiny doses of the liquid. Used in this way, the effects came on in a few minutes and ended within a half-hour. As might be expected, the reactions were highly variable, just as with alcohol. But though there are reports of a few "ether addicts" from this period, most people probably tried the drug only once or twice out of curiosity. A few writers of the time claimed that ether gave them profound insights into the nature of reality and even mystical revelations.* Occasionally, people still experiment with ether, but if they like the effect it gives, they tend to look for other drugs that are less toxic, don't smell as bad, and won't blow up so easily.

*An 1874 book by the American physician Benjamin Paul Blood was titled *The Anesthetic Revelation and the Gist of Philosophy*.

Nitrous oxide is such a drug. A gas with only a faint odor, it is relatively nontoxic, and also nonflammable — although it will support combustion the way oxygen does and should be kept away from flames. Discovered in the late 1700s, nitrous oxide was quickly found to produce interesting changes in consciousness, as well as insensitivity to pain. Oddly enough, no one thought to use it in surgery until after the demonstration of ether anesthesia.

Nitrous oxide is a weaker drug than ether and the other general anesthetics, not producing complete loss of consciousness or anesthesia deep enough for major surgery. Nor is it so strong as to stop respiration. It is widely used in dentistry and minor surgery, however, and many hospital anesthetists like to begin operations by having patients breathe nitrous oxide, then shift to ether and stronger drugs when the patients become totally relaxed and semiconscious.

People have been experimenting with nitrous oxide as a curiosity for the past two hundred years. Its effects, which come on within seconds, last as long as the gas is breathed, then disappear suddenly when it is stopped. Artists, writers, and philosophers have breathed nitrous oxide over and over in pursuit of elusive insights — revelations that seem overpowering under the influence of the gas, but which evaporate as soon as normal consciousness returns. When the English poet laureate Robert Southey tried the gas at a nitrous oxide party in London in the 1790s, he commented afterward that the atmosphere of the highest of all possible heavens was no doubt composed of nitrous oxide.

On the other hand, many others have used nitrous oxide for less spiritual ends, especially to get hilariously intoxicated. The name "laughing gas" comes from a time when traveling medicine shows and carnivals would invite the public to pay a small price for a minute's worth of nitrous oxide. In these rowdy settings, the gas commonly produced silliness and uncontrollable laughter. Often, the laughers would stop in sudden confusion when the effect of the drug came to its abrupt end.

Today, nitrous oxide is available in many dentists' offices. Realizing that people like to get high on it, some dentists give nitrous oxide even for routine procedures such as cleaning teeth. A fair number of tanks of the gas regularly disappear from hospitals and medical supply houses to find their way into the homes of recreational users. Many more people obtain smaller cylinders of the gas from restaurant suppliers, who use it to pressurize instant whipped cream cans. Some people even buy

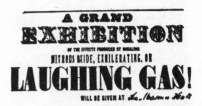

Poster from 1845 advertising a demonstration of the effects of laughing gas (nitrous oxide). (From *Clinical Anesthesia, Nitrous Oxide,* edited by D. W. Eastwood, M.D. Philadelphia: F. A. Davis Co., 1964)

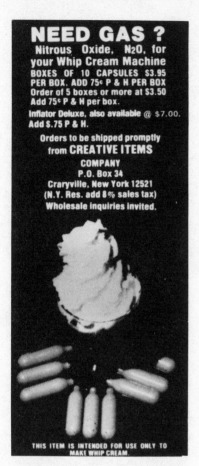
It is unlikely that people responding to this ad were interested in whipped cream; it ran in *High Times*, a magazine of the drug subculture.

cans of instant whipped cream and attempt to get the gas out of the cans without the cream. Balloons of nitrous oxide have been offered for sale at some rock concerts.

Pharmacologically, nitrous oxide is quite safe. Nevertheless, its use in nonmedical settings presents several hazards that users should keep in mind. The only intelligent way to breathe the gas is from balloons. Breathing it directly from pressurized tanks is dangerous for two reasons. First, gas flowing from such tanks is very cold — cold enough to cause frostbite of noses, lips, and vocal cords. Being anesthetized, a user may be unaware of such injuries until too late. Second, because nitrous oxide does not support life, it should be mixed with oxygen if it is to be breathed for more than a few minutes. At private parties, oxygen tanks are rarely supplied, and people have died of asphyxiation by breathing straight nitrous oxide through face masks. The best way to avoid these dangers is to fill balloons from tanks and breathe from the balloons.

Further, nitrous oxide rapidly leads to complete loss of motor control, and anyone who breathes it while standing will soon reel about and fall down. Therefore, it is unwise to try the gas unless one is in a comfortable sitting or lying position. Serious injuries have resulted from people inhaling laughing gas while standing in front of open windows, when driving cars, or when operating machinery. Others have been badly hurt by accidentally pulling heavy tanks of nitrous oxide over onto themselves while intoxicated.

People who breathe nitrous oxide for more than a few minutes at a time may experience nausea, especially if they have just eaten. They may also feel hung over for some time after. In general, however, side effects are few. Some people like laughing gas a great deal and breathe it off and on over months and years. Many of them eventually come to feel that such activity is a waste of time.

Narcotics

The word *narcotic* comes from a Greek word meaning "stupor." Stupor is a state of reduced sensibility that has given rise to our familiar adjective *stupid*. Narcotics are drugs that can produce stupors by depressing brain function, but their depressant action is different from that of sedative-hypnotics or general anesthetics.

The parent of all narcotic drugs is opium, a dark, gummy solid made from the opium poppy. Opium poppies are lovely flowers, probably native to southern Europe and western Asia but now cultivated all over the world. As the flowers wither, the green pods, containing many tiny seeds, begin to ripen and swell. If the pods are allowed to ripen fully, they turn brown and dry, whereupon the edible seeds can be gathered for use in cooking. While still unripe, the pods contain a milky juice that can be collected by letting it ooze from knife cuts. When dried, this juice is crude opium.

One of the oldest of all drugs, opium was used in prehistoric times; the ancient Greeks recognized its pain-relieving properties. Throughout history opium has been an important item of commerce, and in some periods it was the most widely used medical drug.

Opium can be taken by mouth or it can be smoked, but since smoking was unknown in Europe and Asia until Columbus brought news of it from the New World, opium smoking did not exist before 1492. Many oral preparations of opium were made in the past. Two that survive into our own times are paregoric, a dilute tincture of opium combined with camphor, and deodorized tincture of opium, formerly known as laudanum, which is more concentrated.

Crude opium tastes very bitter and contains more than twenty different drugs, of which the most important is morphine. Named for Morpheus, the Greek god of dreams, morphine was isolated from opium in 1803 by a German pharmacist — an event that marked the beginning of the modern era of drug treatment, because it was the first time that an active principle

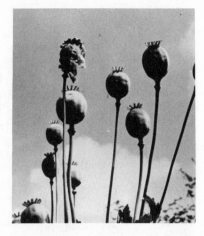

Ripening opium pods. (Jeremy Bigwood)

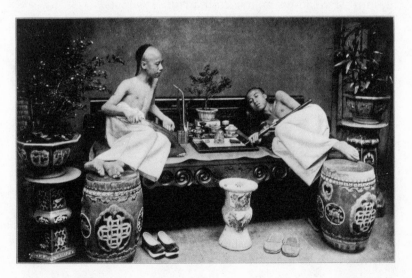

An elegant opium den in Hankow, China, about 1900. (Courtesy of the Swiss Federal Institute of Technology)

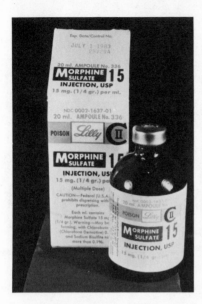

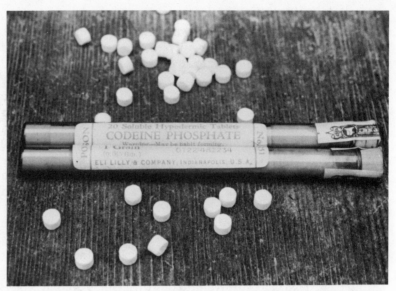

Morphine was the first active principle ever extracted from a drug plant. Its isolation from opium in 1803 marked the beginning of the modern era of drug treatment. (Jeremy Bigwood)

Right: Injectable codeine. (Jeremy Bigwood)

was extracted from a drug plant. Morphine is prepared as a soluble white powder that can be mixed with water and injected into the body. Given by injection, it is a far more powerful and dangerous drug than when taken by mouth. Injection of drugs is relatively recent, dating back only to the invention of the hypodermic syringe in 1853. Interestingly enough, the world's first morphine addict was the wife of the man who came up with that device.

Codeine (methylmorphine) is another natural constituent of opium. More active by mouth than other narcotics, it is a weaker pain reliever than morphine, and doctors frequently prescribe it today as a treatment for moderate pain.

In the late 1800s, chemists began to experiment with variations on molecules of morphine and other compounds of opium. One of the drugs they produced was heroin, a simple derivative of morphine first made available in 1898. Heroin (diacetylmorphine) is more potent than morphine — that is, it produces the same effect in smaller doses — but otherwise the two are very similar. In fact, heroin is promptly converted back into morphine in the body.

Drugs derived from morphine and other opium compounds are called opiates. Today, many hundreds of opiates are known; some are semisynthetic derivatives, like heroin, and others are purely synthetic, like Demerol. In general, all of the opiates produce similar effects. They differ from each other in potency, in duration of action, in how active they are by mouth, and in how much mood change they cause relative to their physical effects. Opiates that are more potent, shorter-acting, and more active by injection also lend themselves more easily to abuse.

The main effects of opium and its derivatives are on the brain and the bowel. In the brain, these drugs cause relief of pain, suppression of the cough center and stimulation of the vomiting center, relaxation, and drowsiness. They may also cause mental clouding and inability to concentrate. Although they may induce sleep, they do not do so as reliably as the sedative-hypnotics. Some people become anxious, restless, and wakeful after taking opiates; others fall into a kind of twilight sleep marked by vivid dreams. Opium and opiates cause the pupils of the eyes to contract, sometimes to tiny pinpoints; they also cause sweating, which can be profuse and uncomfortable. Larger doses often produce nausea, vomiting, and depression of breathing. High doses of opiates, especially by injection, can cause death by stopping respiration, just like other strong depressants.

By paralyzing intestinal muscles, narcotics also lead to constipation, and so are used by doctors to treat diarrhea, particularly when it is accompanied by painful cramps.

In medicine today, narcotics are the main drugs used to treat severe pain. They are also prescribed to control bad coughs. In proper doses, when they are really needed, opiates are safe and extremely effective. Anyone who has experienced the rapid relief of terrible pain by narcotics knows what blessings they can be. By allowing sick and injured people to take their minds off pain, to feel better, to relax and rest, they can also indirectly promote healing. Opium and its derivatives have earned a secure place in treatment over many years of medical experience.

Yet narcotics have generated more fear and argument than any other class of drugs. The reason, of course, is their potential to cause addiction, a problem that was probably recognized even by ancient peoples when the only form available was crude opium from poppies.

Narcotics addiction provides the classic model of drug dependence, and many of our current notions of drug abuse are based on it. For example, the fundamental principle that addiction consists of three features — craving for the drug, tolerance, and withdrawal — developed from observations of opiate addicts. Many popular beliefs about narcotics are untrue, however, and the whole subject is highly contaminated by prejudice and emotion.

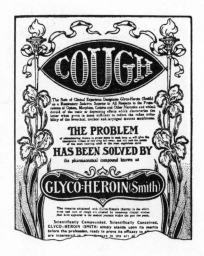

Heroin enjoyed brief popularity as a cough suppressant immediately after its invention. This advertisement appeared in a 1903 medical journal. (© 1903 by the New York Times Company. Reprinted by permission)

There is no question that dependence on narcotics, with physical components, can develop quickly with repeated administration. When medical patients receive morphine by injection every four hours, some degree of dependence can occur in as few as twenty-four hours. If the drug is stopped even after a short period of use, mild withdrawal symptoms may occur — including sweating, nausea, weakness, headache, restlessness, and increased sensitivity to pain.

Tolerance to narcotics also develops rapidly and can reach striking levels. The usual pain-relieving dose of tincture of opium (laudanum) is twenty drops in a glass of water, repeated every four to six hours if necessary. In England in the early 1800s, a number of writers and artists were laudanum addicts with phenomenal habits. The poet Samuel Taylor Coleridge, for example, consumed as much as *two quarts* of laudanum a week. Thomas De Quincey, best known for his *Confessions of an English Opium Eater*, took up to eight thousand drops a day. Such doses would certainly kill nontolerant persons.

There is an important difference between tolerance to narcotics and tolerance to sedative-hypnotics. As noted earlier, tolerance to the active dose of some sedative-hypnotics develops more rapidly than does tolerance to the lethal dose, a process that can — and does — result in fatal accidents. This is not the case with narcotics, however, which makes them safer drugs. Heroin addicts occasionally die of overdoses, but such deaths result from poor quality control in street supplies of the drugs, rather than from the properties of heroin itself.*

Withdrawal from narcotics is also less hazardous than withdrawal from sedative-hypnotics. Alcohol, downers, and even the minor tranquilizers can produce violent withdrawal, marked by convulsions and, sometimes, death. Narcotics withdrawal can be intensely unpleasant, but it is rarely life-threatening.

Also, the physical consequences of long-term narcotics use are minor compared to those of alcohol. People can take opium and opiates every day for years and remain in good health, provided they keep up good habits of hygiene and nutrition. There are many documented cases of opium and morphine addicts who, despite lifelong, heavy habits, survived to ripe old ages, remaining healthy to the end. Thomas De Quincey, for instance, who started taking laudanum for a toothache as a college student, died at seventy-four, still an addict. The worst medical

Laudanum gave me repose, not sleep; but you, I believe, know how divine that repose is, what a spot of enchantment, a green spot of fountains and flowers and trees in the very heart of a waste of sands!
— *Samuel Taylor Coleridge (1772–1834), from a 1798 letter to George Coleridge*

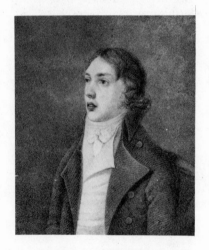

Samuel Taylor Coleridge. (Painting by R. Hancock. Courtesy of the National Portrait Gallery, London)

*For example, an addict used to a certain dose of impure street heroin may buy a packet of the drug that, by accident, hasn't been cut as much as usual; injecting what he thinks is the right dose, he can unwittingly take too much.

effect of regular opiate use is severe and chronic constipation, which can be distressing, but hardly compares to the cirrhosis of the liver, hormonal imbalances, and degeneration of the nervous system so commonly seen in chronic alcoholics.

Some addicts even claim that opiates help them to resist disease. Many heroin users say they don't get colds or other respiratory infections as long as they take their drug. Since the symptoms of heroin withdrawal resemble those of a respiratory flu, it is possible that the drug somehow suppresses this kind of reaction. No one has investigated this claim of addicts; it would make an interesting subject of research.

The strong craving that characterizes opiate addiction has inspired many critics of the drugs to suggest that narcotics destroy the will and moral sense, turning normal people into fiends and degenerates. Actually, cravings for opiates are no different from cravings for alcohol among alcoholics, and they are less strong than cravings for cigarettes, a more addictive drug.

The antisocial behavior of some opiate addicts seems more a function of personality, cultural background, expectation, and setting than of the drugs. Medical patients who become addicted to morphine in hospital settings usually do not conform to stereotypes of addicts, and people who can afford to support opiate habits legally often lead normal lives while also being addicts. There are numerous cases on record of doctors and nurses who were opiate addicts, yet seemed outwardly normal, and fulfilled their professional and social responsibilities.

Apparently, a crucial difference exists between people who become addicted by chance or through medical circumstance, and those who seek out opiates as a means of dealing with life's everyday difficulties. As with other depressants, serious dependence is most likely to develop when people use the drugs to screen out feelings of anxiety, depression, or boredom. Narcotics may be particularly seductive because they insulate people from discomfort and pain, seem to make time pass more rapidly, and create an inner world of security and comfort into which users can retreat, temporarily, from reality and its demands.

In today's world, heroin addiction has reached epidemic proportions. It swallows up many people, especially the young, in unproductive lives of great hardship and cost to themselves and society, and is rightly a cause for serious concern. It is not only the downtrodden poor of urban ghettos who become heroin addicts, but the children of all social and economic classes and many of their parents as well.

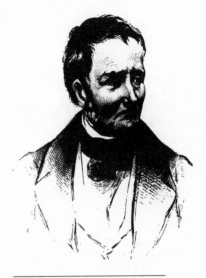

Thomas De Quincey (1785–1859), the Victorian writer, author of *Confessions of an English Opium Eater*. (Fitz Hugh Ludlow Memorial Library)

Junk is not a kick. It is a way of life.
— *William S. Burroughs, from his novel* Junky *(1953)*

When ordinary people look at heroin addicts, what they mostly see are victims of grinding social forces. Visible addicts tend to be in trouble, involved with crime, in poor health, purposeless, psychologically damaged, unhappy, and unable to get out of their grim predicaments. It is impossible, however, to tell which of these conditions is due to heroin itself, and which to society's blunders in trying to control the abuse of drugs.

Heroin is often portrayed as the very worst of all possible drugs, a "devil drug," always productive of evil and somehow especially dangerous. In reality it isn't very different from morphine, an accepted medical drug. Heroin is strictly illegal in the United States; even doctors cannot obtain it to use on patients. It is legal in England, however, where doctors do use it, sometimes with good results. Because it is more potent than morphine, it is sometimes a better pain reliever in small doses for people who are too sensitive to the nauseating effect of morphine.

By making heroin illegal, a society ensures that its heroin addicts will all be criminals. It is clear that our drug laws have done nothing to discourage young people from becoming addicts. There are as many addicts as ever, and the kinds of addiction are worse than before those laws were passed. Prohibition of opiates has directly spawned an ugly criminal underworld that supplies heroin to addicts at grossly inflated prices: up to $200 a gram for material of questionable purity* that may be cut with substances more hazardous than the drug itself. Addicts with habits costing several hundred dollars a day are forced to resort to daily criminal activity in order to avoid the unpleasant symptoms of withdrawal.

It seems obvious that many of the worst features of heroin addiction are due to this social situation rather than to the pharmacological effects of opiates. When you have to come up with several hundred dollars a day to buy a drug you must have to avoid feeling sick, you aren't likely to eat well, sleep regularly, or live in healthy surroundings. Heroin addicts are usually unproductive because they have little time for anything but scoring heroin and then nodding out in isolation.

The aspects of addiction that are attributable directly to heroin have to do with the high potency of the drug, its short duration of action, and the tendency for people to use it intravenously.† Heroin can be smoked (mixed with tobacco or mari-

*Pure heroin's street value is $500 a gram.

†The health problems associated with intravenous drug use are discussed in Chapter 12.

juana); snuffed up the nose; or injected under the skin, into a muscle, or into a vein. By any of these routes it is much more powerful than by mouth. Oddly enough, most people who try heroin for the first time, by whatever route, don't find it pleasant; more often than not, they experience little besides nausea, sweating, and a general feeling of discomfort. After a few doses, however — particularly when it is injected directly into the bloodstream — some people experience an intense "rush" of good feeling that lasts for a few minutes, and then become drowsy.

To hear heroin addicts talk about the intensity of this rush is both fascinating and frightening. Some say it is the most pleasurable sensation they have ever felt, much more powerful than orgasm. People who get this experience from "mainlining" heroin — not all do — find it hard to appreciate other kinds of highs, especially nondrug highs, which tend to be more subtle. The power of the heroin rush to make people uninterested in other experiences and totally committed to heroin is so overwhelming as to be an argument against ever trying the drug at all. One junkie expressed this sentiment in a much-quoted line: "It's so good, don't even try it once."

Nonintravenous heroin doesn't give nearly as intense a rush and so is less addicting. People who snort heroin can do so off and on for long periods of time without becoming strongly addicted. Even people who inject it subcutaneously ("skin-popping") can sometimes avoid full-blown dependence, being able to confine their use of the drug to occasional sprees. There is no question that some users can mainline heroin only once in a while, usually shooting the drug only in certain situations — to reduce anxiety in personal relationships, for example, or to boost their confidence before a public performance, or to feel good at weekend parties. In street jargon, this sort of occasional use of heroin is known as "chipping," and it seems that some lucky individuals remain successful chippers over months and even years. Unfortunately, a high percentage of chippers eventually go on to become addicts, so the practice is risky. Most junkies began as chippers, and many never thought they would become addicts.

Once physical dependence develops, however, the need to avoid withdrawal becomes a powerful motive for taking more of the drug. Three to eight hours after his last dose, a heroin addict will begin to feel sick, and unless he takes another fix these feelings will grow more and more intense.

It's too bad that heroin has become the most popular street opiate. Whole opium, when eaten, is a much safer drug — less

There's nothing like a heroin rush. I started shooting heroin when I was fourteen. It's just the most intense, wonderful feeling. I was always interested in getting high. One of my favorite ways when I was little was rolling down big hills. I did it over and over. Heroin has caused me a lot of problems. I'm scared of withdrawal, but I know I have to do it. I'm also interested in meditation and things like that, but I worry that I will always be tempted to feel the heroin rush again, because nothing else I've tried comes close to it.
— seventeen-year-old woman, patient in a private addiction treatment center

concentrated, longer acting, and easier to form stable relationships with. Because it is a gummy solid, it cannot be injected directly into the bloodstream, and though people can certainly become addicted to it — as they did in England and America in the 1800s — the risk is much less. Taking opium orally doesn't give a rush, and high doses cause unpleasant nausea, encouraging users to moderate their intake. Smoking opium puts drugs into the blood and brain more directly and has a higher potential for abuse.

Many junkies are as addicted to giving themselves intravenous injections as they are to the effects of heroin. Some of them experiment with shooting other drugs, and some combine other drugs with their heroin. For instance, some addicts mix heroin and cocaine into a "speedball" that gives an intense euphoric effect. Of course, this practice is dangerous, much more so than combinations of stimulants and depressants taken by mouth.

Treatments of narcotics addiction are not very satisfactory. The physical component of an opiate habit can be broken fairly easily by withdrawing people gradually and treating symptoms as they develop. As with cigarette addiction, however, the relapse rate is very high, and junkies often go back to being junkies even after being drug-free for months or years.

Heroin maintenance — that is, supplying addicts with pure, legal heroin in some sort of supervised setting — has been proposed as a possible treatment, but our society, unwilling to abandon its prohibitionist mentality, has been unwilling to try it, even as an experiment. Instead, it has supported maintenance with methadone, a synthetic opiate that is active by mouth and has a long duration of effect. Oral methadone is an addicting narcotic but gives little euphoria. It does block the effect of heroin, however, and so may reduce a junkie's motivation to shoot heroin. Some addicts sign into methadone programs only to take a break from the street scene; after a time, they go right back to their old ways. Other addicts, if they are highly motivated, can use methadone programs to help them break their heroin habits once and for all.

The main advantage of methadone maintenance is that it is better than leading a criminal life. The real problem with it is that it doesn't go to the root of addiction. Nor does it show heroin users how to get high in more natural, less restricting ways. It offers them no help with the problems that led them to abuse heroin in the first place. All it does is substitute one narcotic for another; the addict remains an addict, albeit in a less destructive way.

No matter how you look at it, heroin addiction limits personal freedom. Like a cigarette addict, the junkie cannot go anywhere or do anything without thinking about where his next fix is coming from. Unlike the cigarette addict, he cannot buy his drug for a reasonable price at the corner store, and he will become really sick if he cannot get it.

Nowadays, heroin use is becoming more and more common — invading affluent and respectable segments of society. In some circles it is fashionable to try heroin or use it occasionally, particularly by means of "chasing the dragon," the practice of heating brown Asian heroin on tinfoil and inhaling the vapors. Though the medical dangers of heroin have certainly been exaggerated, the risk of addiction is real.

If you do not try heroin, you will not use it. If you do not use it, you will never become addicted.

Many questions about opiate addiction remain unanswered. How much of it is biochemical and how much is psychological? Opiate molecules interact with special receptor sites on nerve cells in the brain. Might addiction be the result of suppression of the brain's own opiatelike molecules, the endorphins? Why do some people who try opiates find them so compelling that they go on to become addicts, while others do not? Is this a matter of differences in brain chemistry, or differences in personality? Unfortunately, the answers are still hidden.

Given these uncertainties, it is impossible to say who is at greatest risk of addiction and who is not. There is no assurance that you will not become an addict once you start using opiates regularly, and no way of taking the drugs so as to protect yourself from that possibility. Furthermore, once addiction develops, there is no reliable method of breaking it.

*The first opiate I ever took was codeine . . . It made me feel right for the first time in my life . . . I never felt right from as far back as I can remember, and I was always trying different ways to change how I felt. I used lots of drugs, but none of them really did it for me. Codeine was a revelation, and I've been an opiate user ever since . . . Opiates have caused me lots of trouble, but what they do for my head is worth it.
— thirty-four-year-old woman, rock singer*

Precautions About Narcotics

1. Opium and its derivatives are powerful drugs that should be reserved for treating severe physical pain and discomfort.
2. Taking narcotics to reduce anxiety or depression, or just to feel good in the absence of physical pain, can easily lead to habitual use and addiction.
3. Never inject a narcotic into the body for nonmedical purposes.
4. If you ever try a narcotic intravenously and feel overwhelming pleasure, *never repeat it.*
5. If you begin to use narcotics regularly, by any method, and think you can avoid going on to intravenous use and addiction, remember: most junkies thought that, too.

Suggested Reading

Margaret O. Hyde's *Alcohol: Drink or Drug?* (New York: McGraw-Hill, 1974) is a good book written for adolescent readers. Berton Roueché's *The Neutral Spirit: A Portrait of Alcohol* (Boston: Little, Brown, 1960) is a well-written account of the uses of alcohol from ancient times to the present. A more technical book is *Under the Influence: A Guide to the Myths and Realities of Alcoholism* by James R. Milam and Katherine Ketcham (Seattle: Madrona, 1981). An account of writers with alcohol problems is Donald Newlove's *Those Drinking Days: Myself and Other Writers* (New York: Horizon Press, 1981). Evelyn Waugh's *Brideshead Revisited* (Boston: Little, Brown, 1945; reprinted in paper, 1979) describes the evolution of an English alcoholic. For a view of the use and abuse of alcohol on this side of the Atlantic, see *The Alcohol Republic: An American Tradition* by W. J. Rorabaugh (New York: Oxford University Press, 1979). The connection between violent crime and alcohol is explored in *The Crocodile Man: A Case of Brain Chemistry and Criminal Violence* by André Mayer and Michael Wheeler (Boston: Houghton Mifflin, 1982).

Several excellent films dramatize the problem of alcoholism. One classic is *The Lost Weekend*, about an alcoholic writer played by Ray Milland. *Days of Wine and Roses,* starring Jack Lemmon and Lee Remick, is an agonizing portrait of a pair of alcoholics whose lives are destroyed by drinking. An equally moving account of a person ravaged by alcohol (and other drugs) is *The Rose*, based on the life of the late rock singer Janis Joplin. *Only When I Laugh*, starring Marsha Mason as an alcoholic mother, takes a somewhat more humorous view of the problem drinker.

One of the few resource books on downers is *Barbiturates: Their Use and Misuse* by Donald R. Wesson and David E. Smith (New York: Human Sciences Press, 1977); both authors are physicians. A novel in which downers figure prominently is Jacqueline Susann's *Valley of the Dolls* (New York: Bantam, 1967), which was also made into a movie. The minor tranquilizers and their manufacturers are strongly criticized in *The Tranquilizing of America: Pill Popping and the American Way of Life* by Richard Hughes and Robert Brewin (New York: Harcourt Brace Jovanovich, 1979). One woman's personal story of addiction to Valium is told in *I'm Dancing as Fast as I Can* by Barbara Gordon (New York: Harper & Row, 1979), recently adapted for the screen.

The best information on general anesthetics will be found in *Licit and Illicit Drugs* by Edward M. Brecher and the editors of *Consumer Reports* (Boston: Little, Brown, 1972), an excellent book that also has a good section on sedative-hypnotics. A short but entertaining and informative book on nitrous oxide is *Laughing Gas (Nitrous Oxide)* edited by Michael Sheldin and David Wallechinsky, with Saunie Salyer (Berkeley, California: And/Or Press, 1973).

The history of opium dating back to ancient times is presented in *Flowers in the Blood: The Story of Opium* by Dean Latimer and Jeff Goldberg (New York: Franklin Watts, 1981). Thomas De Quincey's *Confessions of an English Opium Eater*, first published in 1821, is available in a modern edition (New York: Penguin, 1971). *The Opium Eater: A Life of Thomas De Quincey* by Grevel Lindop (New York: Taplinger, 1982) is a fascinating biography of the man who became world-famous at the age of thirty-six, when his *Confessions* appeared. A number of novels concern opium, among them Charles Dickens's last work, *The Mystery of Edwin Drood*, written in 1870 and concluded by Leon Garfield (New York: Pantheon, 1980), and Wilkie Collins's classic from 1873, *The Moonstone* (New York: Penguin, 1966). Louisa May Alcott wrote a short story about opium: "A Marble Woman: *or*, The Mysterious Model," collected in *Plots and Counterplots: More Unknown Thrillers of Louisa May Alcott*, edited by Madeleine Stern (New York: William Morrow, 1976).

A readable and factual book on heroin is Richard Ashley's *Heroin: The Myths and the Facts* (New York: St. Martin's Press, 1972). A newer book that suggests how society might reduce the destructiveness of heroin abuse by legalizing the drug for medical purposes and allowing doctors to take control of it is *The Heroin Solution* by Arnold S. Trebach (New Haven: Yale University Press, 1982). Trebach is a law professor and expert on drugs, crime, and justice. His analysis of the heroin problem is reasoned, persuasive, and not sensational.

A number of creative writers have left us autobiographical records of their involvement with opium and opiates. One of the best is *Opium: The Diary of a Cure* by the French artist, writer, and film maker Jean Cocteau (translated by Margaret Crosland and Sinclair Road; New York: Grove Press, 1980). Another is *Junky* by William S. Burroughs (New York: Penguin, 1977), which was first published in 1953 under the pseudonym William Lee. Aleister Crowley's *Diary of a Drug Fiend* (New York: Samuel Weiser, 1970) is an autobiographical novel about two English aristocrats addicted to heroin and cocaine. Alexander

Trocchi's novel *Cain's Book* (New York: Grove Press, 1960) is a vivid picture of the often nightmarish world of the heroin addict. One of the best-known novels about heroin addiction is Nelson Algren's 1949 book *The Man with the Golden Arm* (New York: Penguin, 1977); it was made into a popular movie starring Frank Sinatra. Eugene O'Neill's play *Long Day's Journey into Night,* also made into a movie, is a harrowing account of his mother's addiction to morphine. More recent movies dealing with opiates are *McCabe and Mrs. Miller* and *Christine F,* a West German film based on the real case of a teen-age prostitute and heroin addict.

8

Psychedelics, or Hallucinogens

T HE PLANTS AND CHEMICALS discussed in this chapter are some of the most colorful and controversial of all drugs. Some users have recommended them enthusiastically, claiming they are keys to understanding our minds and the origins of religious feelings. Many nonusers are fearful of them, regarding them as dangerous agents capable of driving people to insanity and suicide.

So heated is the debate over whether these drugs are good or evil that it's hard even to find a neutral name for them. When they first came to the attention of scientists in Europe and America in the 1950s, they were called *psychotomimetics*, based on the belief that they made people temporarily insane. (Psychiatrists now recognize that important differences exist between psychosis and the states induced by these drugs.)

Many of the subjects who volunteered for the early research with these chemicals liked their effects very much. Unlike the doctors studying the drugs, they thought of them in positive ways and frequently wanted to repeat the experiences with friends outside laboratories. As this group of devotees grew in number, they sought a more favorable name for the substances and came up with *psychedelics*, a word coined from Greek roots meaning "mind manifesting." The implication is that psychedelic drugs can develop unused potentials of the human mind.

At about the same time, the medical profession was using the term *hallucinogens* for the same compounds, meaning "causers of hallucinations." Since hallucinations are common symptoms of schizophrenia, this term carries the suggestion that the drug state is abnormal and unhealthy. The battle over names goes on. We will use *psychedelics* and *hallucinogens* interchangeably.

The substances in this class probably have the lowest potential for abuse of any psychoactive drugs. In purely medical terms, they may be the safest of all known drugs. Even in huge overdose, psychedelics do not kill, and some people take them frequently all their lives without suffering physical damage or dependence. In the right hands they can bring about dramatic cures of both physical and mental illnesses. Yet these same drugs can cause the most frightening experiences imaginable, leaving long-lasting psychological scars.

Primitive people discovered hallucinogenic plants and began using them long before recorded history. Though many such plants exist, most are concentrated in North and South America, with heaviest use occurring among Indians of Mexico and Colombia. Very few natural psychedelics are native to the Old World and there is little traditional use of them there. The main Old World psychedelic is a plant called iboga, whose root is made into a drink consumed in religious rituals by a few tribes of west Africa.

By contrast, hundreds of tribes of New World Indians use dozens of different hallucinogenic plants in tropical areas of North and South America. Among these people, the use of hallucinogens is tied to native practices of magic, medicine, and religion, particularly to the primitive religion called shamanism. In shamanism, special individuals, or shamans, attempt to control the forces of good and evil within the tribal community by communicating between the human world and the spirit world. To contact the spirit world, shamans put themselves in altered states of consciousness, often by consuming hallucinogenic plants. Shamans (or medicine men) also take psychedelics to see visions, and they use the visions to locate missing persons or lost objects and to diagnose illness. They often treat illness by administering psychedelics to sick people. In certain tribes, many people consume the plants at the same time in group vision-seeking rituals.

Most hallucinogenic plants taste bitter and cause nausea, vomiting, or other unpleasant physical symptoms at the onset of their effects. Then they induce unusual states of consciousness and fantastic visions seen with the eyes closed. However, visions and other sensory changes seem to come from taking these plants in particular ways, and are by no means invariable occurrences. Indians who believe in the importance of visions and who eat hallucinogenic plants at night in front of fires while chanting and praying under the direction of skilled shamans are much more likely to have visions than non-Indians who eat the same plants for purely recreational purposes. In fact, the mental effects of psychedelics are completely dependent on set and setting — on who takes them and why, on where and how.

Physical effects, on the other hand, are more constant, because all of the hallucinogenic drugs have some common pharmacological actions. All of them are strong stimulants, for instance, causing increased brain activity and wakefulness. And they all stimulate the sympathetic nervous system, usually causing widely dilated eyes, a sensation of butterflies in the stomach, and feelings of cold in the extremities. The various psychedelics differ mainly in their duration of action and how fast their effects come on.

These substances fall into two broad chemical families. The first, called indoles, contain a molecular structure known as the indole ring and are related to hormones made in the brain by the pineal gland. The drugs in the second family lack the indole ring; instead, they closely resemble molecules of adrenaline and the amphetamines.

Indole Hallucinogens

LSD (Lysergic Acid Diethylamide, Acid, LSD-25)

LSD is the most famous of the psychedelics, probably the one that has been tried by the most people. It is a semisynthetic drug, not found in nature. A Swiss chemist first made it in a laboratory in 1938 from lysergic acid, a chemical in ergot, the fungus that attacks cereal grains, especially rye. At the time, he was interested in developing medical drugs from compounds in ergot. In 1943 the same chemist accidently consumed some LSD and so discovered its psychoactivity. Beginning in the late 1940s, the Swiss pharmaceutical company he worked for supplied LSD as a research drug to doctors and hospitals throughout the world.

LSD is one of the most potent drugs known, producing its effects in doses as small as 25 micrograms. (A microgram is one millionth of a gram, and there are 28 grams in an ounce. An average postage stamp weighs about 60,000 micrograms.) An LSD trip lasts ten to twelve hours.

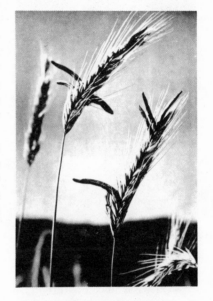

Ergot growing on rye. The hard, black spurs of fungus replace the grains and contain a number of drugs, including lysergic acid, the precursor of LSD. (Sandoz, Ltd., Basel, Switzerland)

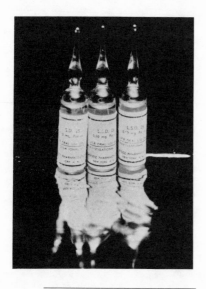

Pharmaceutical LSD-25.
(Jeremy Bigwood)

Throughout the 1950s, LSD remained mostly in the hands of researchers, especially psychiatrists. But many people who tried the drug found it so interesting that they publicized its effects and began taking it on their own. At first, most of the LSD in circulation was pure pharmaceutical material from the Swiss laboratory that originally made it. In the 1960s, when the psychedelic movement started in Europe and America, black-market LSD began to appear.

For the most part, people who took LSD in the early days had pleasant trips. They talked about experiencing powerful feelings of love, mystical oneness with all things, union with God, and a deeper understanding of themselves. Some described vivid sensory changes they enjoyed, such as seeing flowers breathe, objects shimmer with energy, and mosaic patterns appear on all surfaces. Such descriptions made other people, especially young people, eager to try the drug for themselves.

From the very first, however, it was apparent that not everyone who takes LSD has a good time. Some people had bad trips: they became anxious and panicky, afraid they were losing their minds and would be unable to return to ordinary reality. They almost always did return, when the drug wore off twelve hours later, but some of them remained depressed and anxious for days afterward, and a few had lasting psychological problems.

When people are panicked they often behave in violent and irrational ways. In the 1960s some bad trips on LSD may have led to accidents and suicides. Even though these cases were exceptional, the media seized on them and made it seem as if LSD were a new drug menace that threatened to turn teen-agers into lunatics.

DOONESBURY

by Garry Trudeau

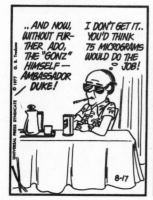

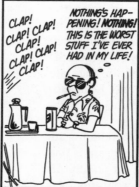

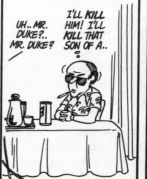

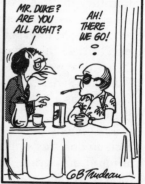

Bad trips are more likely to occur when people take LSD in inappropriate settings, especially if they have never taken it before and if they take high doses. Throughout the 1960s black-market LSD was unreliable, sometimes contaminated with other drugs, and since not many people were familiar with the effects of LSD, bad trips were common. By the 1970s, bad trips were rare, not because fewer people were taking the drug, but because people had learned how to use it intelligently. They took reasonable doses in good settings (such as a familiar room or a peaceful field in the country), with friends who knew what to expect.

Street LSD comes in a bewildering array of forms, from small tablets of all colors and tiny transparent gelatin chips ("windowpane") to pieces of paper soaked in solutions of the drug or stamped with ink designs containing it. The windowpane and paper forms are likely to be the purest, since they are too small to contain contaminants.

Despite loud arguments and much bad publicity about the medical dangers of LSD in the 1970s, there is no evidence that it damages chromosomes, injures the brain, or causes any other physical harm.*

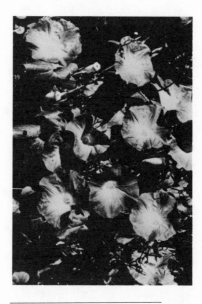

Morning-glory. (R. G. Wasson)

Morning-Glory Seeds

The closest substance to LSD that occurs in nature is a chemical called ergine, or lysergic acid amide, found in the seeds of certain morning-glories. Indians in southern Mexico were eating morning-glory seeds for ritual purposes before the Spanish arrived, and some still use them today.

Not all the varieties of morning-glories available from seed companies are psychoactive. Of those that are, the best known are Heavenly Blue (with large blue flowers), Pearly Gates (white), Wedding Bells (pink), and Flying Saucers (blue with white stripes).

Because the concentration of LSD-like activity in the seeds of these plants is low, it takes a great many to produce a noticeable psychedelic effect, even up to several hundred, or a whole cupful. The seeds, which have hard, indigestible coats, must be cracked or ground up to release the drug. Also, they seem to be mildly toxic, frequently causing nausea, vomiting, and other uncomfortable side effects. For these reasons they are not popular; even the Mexican Indians who use morning-glory seeds re-

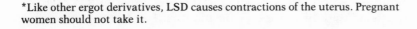

*Like other ergot derivatives, LSD causes contractions of the uterus. Pregnant women should not take it.

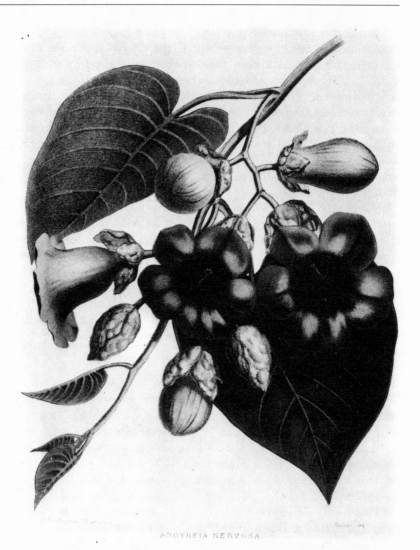

ARGYREIA NERVOSA

Hawaiian Baby Woodrose (a species of morning-glory, *Argyreia nervosa*). (From *Familiar Indian Flowers* by Lena Lowis, London, 1881. Courtesy of Dr. Otto Solbrig, Gray Herbarium, Harvard University. Photograph by John Lupo)

gard them as a back-up psychedelic, taking them only when they can't get the hallucinogenic mushrooms they prefer.

One species of morning-glory that is stronger than others is the Hawaiian Baby Woodrose, a creeping plant that covers many Hawaiian beaches and whose flowers are often dried and sold by florists. A dozen of the large, hard seeds will produce a strong intoxication, but they, too, frequently make people feel sick.

Devotees of psychedelics say that morning-glory seeds are definitely second-rate, producing too much discomfort relative to effects they like. Another problem is that many commercial

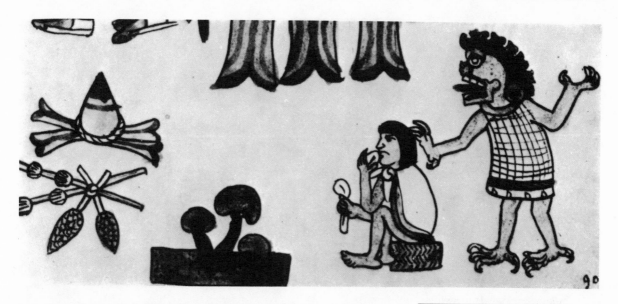

morning-glory seeds are now dipped in poisons to discourage people from eating them — sometimes without any caution to the buyer.

Mushrooms (Magic Mushrooms, Psilocybin)

Mushrooms are the most important natural psychedelics of southern Mexico, used in ceremonies so sacred that Indians carefully concealed them from Europeans until the present century. It wasn't until the 1950s that descriptions of Mexican mushrooms came to the attention of the world. Soon after, botanists began to identify the mushrooms in use, and chemists found that their psychoactive properties came from psilocybin, an indole hallucinogen similar to LSD but with a shorter duration of action: four to six hours.

Mexican mushroom ceremonies are conducted by shamans, usually women, and are held for purposes of treating illness, solving problems, foreseeing the future in visions, and putting people in contact with the supernatural world. They take place at night, by candlelight, and today are curious blends of shamanism and Roman Catholic ritual.

For some years, scientists believed that mushrooms containing psilocybin grew only in southern Mexico, and during the late 1960s and early 1970s thousands of people, mostly from Europe and North America, traveled there to take magic mushrooms in remote Indian villages. For a time, several Swiss pharmaceutical companies manufactured pure psilocybin, supply-

In this drawing from an Aztec manuscript of the sixteenth century, a man eats a pair of sacred mushrooms while a god stands behind him. Three more mushrooms grow in front of him. (Courtesy of the Biblioteca Medicea Laurenziana)

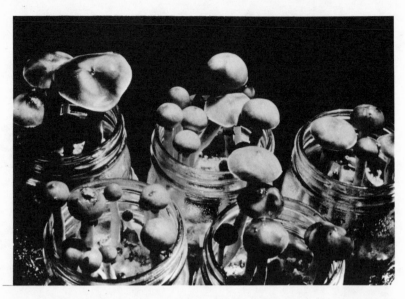

Psilocybe cubensis growing in cultivation on grain. (Jeremy Bigwood)

ing it to researchers. As with LSD, some of this material eventually found its way to the street, but underground chemists never manufactured it because the synthesis is too costly.

As natural substances with a reputation for producing interesting experiences and fewer bad trips than LSD, magic mushrooms have been in great demand on the black market. For a long time they were unavailable, though unscrupulous dealers often sold ordinary supermarket mushrooms laced with LSD and other drugs at high prices to unsuspecting customers.

Since the late 1970s this situation has changed. In the first place, psilocybin mushrooms have been found in great numbers in many parts of the world. One of the principal species, called *Psilocybe cubensis,* is a large mushroom that grows in cow pastures in warm climates. It occurs in Southeast Asia, in Central and South America, all along the Gulf Coast of the United States, and in many southeastern states. More than a dozen species of psychoactive mushrooms grow in fields and woods of the Pacific Northwest. Some grow in Europe as well. In certain areas, the mushrooms are so abundant that collectors can easily gather enough for sale as well as for their own use.

Needless to say, collecting wild mushrooms of any sort requires knowledge and practice, because some mushrooms are very poisonous. No one should attempt to pick magic mushrooms without knowing how to recognize them.

Psilocybin mushrooms can also be cultivated. Although growing mushrooms from spores is much harder than growing green plants from seeds, many people have mastered the technique. *Psilocybe cubensis* is the easiest variety to grow; in recent years, kits that include spores of the mushrooms have been widely sold through the mail and in stores. Since the spores don't contain psilocybin, they aren't illegal. Taking advantage of this loophole in the law, thousands of people have started producing and distributing magic mushrooms. Real, unadulterated mushrooms are now easily obtainable on the black market.

Both wild and cultivated mushrooms vary greatly in potency. One medium-sized mushroom of a potent strain may give the same effect as twenty of a mild strain. It is important, therefore, to get advice on potency and dosages before eating mushrooms in order to avoid unpleasant effects from too high doses.

Many wild mushrooms are hard to digest raw, and some are mildly toxic until they are cooked. Psychedelic mushrooms may taste better and are less likely to cause discomfort if they are dried or lightly cooked before being eaten. Still, mushrooms are generally easier to take than the other hallucinogenic plants. One reason many people prefer mushrooms to other psychedelics is their ease of consumption. Another is that the effects are shorter, usually ending after six hours, and therefore are less demanding on the body. People usually feel sluggish the day after taking LSD or other long-acting psychedelics. This is less common with mushrooms.*

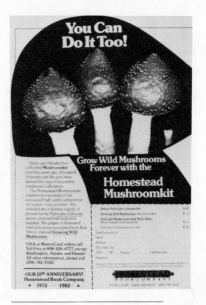

(Copyright © 1982 Homestead Book Company)

Ibogaine

Ibogaine is the active principle of the African hallucinogenic plant iboga. Though the iboga root is almost unknown outside Africa, the pure drug can be made synthetically and sometimes appears on the black market. It is a long-acting psychedelic resembling LSD in effect, but it is an even stronger stimulant. Africans who drink iboga in all-night ceremonies that include vigorous dancing may stay up the next day and night until the stimulation wears off. Eventually they fall into a deep sleep.

DMT (Dimethyltryptamine)

DMT is the drug responsible for the hallucinogenic properties of several plants used by South American Indians. It is a simple chemical closely resembling certain hormones made in the

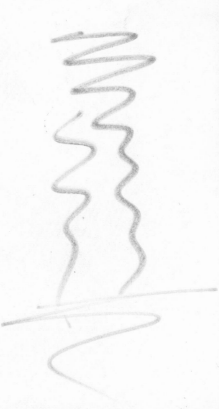

---

*Amanita muscaria, the bright-red fly agaric (mushroom) with white dots on the cap, is not a true hallucinogen. It is discussed in Chapter 10, along with other deliriant drugs.

brain, and it is likely that the brain also produces DMT itself. DMT may be our own endogenous psychedelic. It is a compound easily made in laboratories as well; in the 1960s synthetic DMT was sold in quantity on the black market.

DMT is peculiar among the psychedelics in that it cannot be taken by mouth; an enzyme in the stomach breaks it down before it can enter the bloodstream. Indians who use DMT-containing plants often prepare them as powdered snuffs. Users of the isolated, black-market chemical either smoke it or, less frequently, inject it intramuscularly.

A typical DMT snuff of South America is yopo, used by tribes of the Amazonian forests. It is made from the resin of a huge jungle tree, cooked down, dried, and pounded into a fine powder which the men blow forcefully into each other's noses through long tubes. Taken in this way, yopo causes a very intense intoxication beginning within seconds but lasting only thirty minutes or less. While under its influence, Indians dance, sing, and see visions of gods and spirits.

South American Indians using a DMT-containing snuff. (R. E. Schultes)

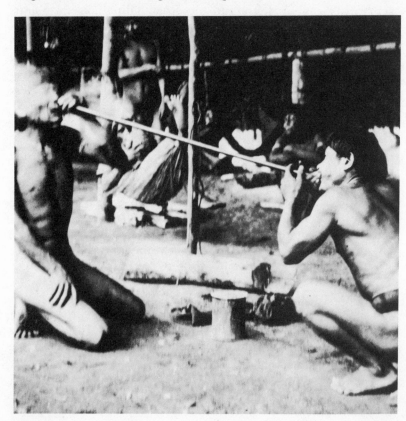

Black-market DMT is usually a brown solid that smells like mothballs; users place tiny bits of it in the ends of joints made with marijuana, mint, or oregano in order to smoke it. Sometimes, a single inhalation of such a joint will be sufficient to initiate a five- to ten-minute trip of remarkable intensity. The effect may begin before a person can remove the joint from his lips and usually reaches its peak within the first minute. Some users lose all awareness of their surroundings, being overwhelmed by visual hallucinations. Fans of DMT say it gives an ultimate psychedelic rush; needless to say, this experience can be quite frightening to someone unprepared for it.

After fifteen minutes, the strong effects subside, and after thirty minutes users again feel normal. Because of its short duration of action, DMT is known as the businessman's trip. It is a good example of the correlation between route of administration, duration of action, and intensity of effect. Short-acting drugs, introduced directly into the bloodstream by smoking or injection, tend to give "rushes" — sudden, dramatic changes in consciousness. Some people are especially fascinated by drug rushes, and, as noted in the section on narcotics, the pursuit of a rush can be the basis of addictive use.

That addiction to DMT is unknown is due to the rapid development of tolerance to its interesting effects. When smoked regularly, it soon becomes ineffective.

All of the psychedelics share this characteristic. The body develops rapid tolerance to them, so that if you try to take them often, you do not get the results you want. Even people who really like these drugs don't take them every day, and most users save them for special occasions.

Yagé (Ayahuasca, Caapi)

Yagé (pronounced yah-HAY) is a strong psychedelic drink made from a woody vine of the Amazon forests. Indians pound up lengths of the vine with stones, then cook them in water for several hours, sometimes adding other plants to heighten the effect. They use the drink in all-night vision-seeking rituals with shamans or in large tribal ceremonies, such as coming-of-age rites for adolescent boys. The plant owes most of its activity to harmaline, a drug rarely seen on the black market. Yagé first causes intense vomiting and diarrhea, and then a more relaxed and dreamy state than that produced by LSD; it lasts from six to ten hours. Indians say the spirit of the vine enters their bodies and makes them see visions of jungles and jungle animals, especially jaguars. Also, the drug is supposed to enable them to see

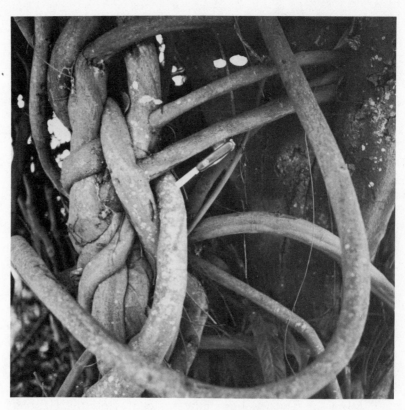

Yagé growing in the jungle in Colombia. The woody vine is the source of a psychedelic drink. (R. E. Schultes)

the future and communicate telepathically over great distances. Seeing visions on yagé, as with other psychedelics, depends very much on set and setting.

Curiously enough, the plant most commonly added to yagé in making the drink is a leaf containing DMT. Indians say the addition makes for better and brighter visions. When scientists first learned of this practice, they dismissed it as useless on the grounds that DMT is destroyed in the stomach. Further research has now shown that harmaline inactivates the enzyme that destroys DMT. Combined with yagé, therefore, DMT becomes orally active, and in this form it is a longer acting, less intense drug that doesn't produce a rush.

How did Indians discover this remarkable combination of plants? Anthropologists and botanists say they did so by trial and error. Given the number of plants in the Amazonian jungles, that would mean a great deal of trial and error. The Indians themselves say they were inspired by visions — that the spirit of yagé showed them the other leaves and the method of cooking the two together.

Hallucinogens Related to Adrenaline and Amphetamines

Indole hallucinogens make people feel high very rapidly. Typically, their effects begin in twenty to forty minutes and reach a peak within the first hour or two. The drugs in this second family of psychedelics may also be felt quickly, but their onset is more gradual, reaching a peak after several hours. Some users find them less "electric" than LSD and its relatives, although in high doses the adrenaline relatives are more toxic than the indoles.

Peyote and Mescaline

Peyote is a small, spineless cactus with white, hairy tufts; it is native to the Rio Grande Valley in southern Texas and north-central Mexico. The tops of the cactus, cut off at ground level, dry into peyote "buttons" that retain their potency for a long time.

Some Indians in Mexico have used peyote since before recorded history, making long pilgrimages to the desert to collect it, then eating it in elaborate ceremonies. When the Spanish conquered Mexico, the Roman Catholic Church tried to stamp out peyote use, calling it sinful and diabolic, but to no avail. In the late 1800s the use of peyote spread northward to Indians in the United States, who invented new rituals around it. As it moved north, peyote became even more popular; Indians of the midwestern plains organized a new religion based on it and helped spread its use all the way to Canada.

Not surprisingly, the explosion of this psychedelic movement among Indians generated intense opposition by non-Indians. Churches and government agencies charged that peyote made Indians crazy and violent; stories circulated of Indian men who, upon eating the cactus, axed helpless victims to death, while Indian women under its influence supposedly ripped off their clothes in sexual frenzies. The similarity of the early peyote stories to those told about other psychoactive drugs is striking. (If there were high-rise tipis, newspapers would doubtless have reported peyote-crazed Indians jumping out of them, thinking they could fly.) The very same charges have been made about LSD, marijuana, heroin, cocaine, and PCP. Rarely have they had any basis in fact.

In response to official efforts to suppress the use of peyote, Indians organized formal churches and fought in courts for their right to eat the cactus. The Native American Church began in

My first vivid show of mescal colour effects came quickly. I saw the stars, and then, of a sudden, here and there delicate floating films of colour — usually delightful neutral purples and pinks. These came and went — now here, now there. Then an abrupt rush of countless points of white light swept across the field of view, as if the unseen millions of the Milky Way were to flow a sparkling river before the eye. In a minute this was over and the field was dark. Then I began to see zigzag lines of very bright colours . . .
— from an essay by Dr. S. Weir Mitchell (1829–1914), an American physician and novelist who drank an extract of peyote in 1896

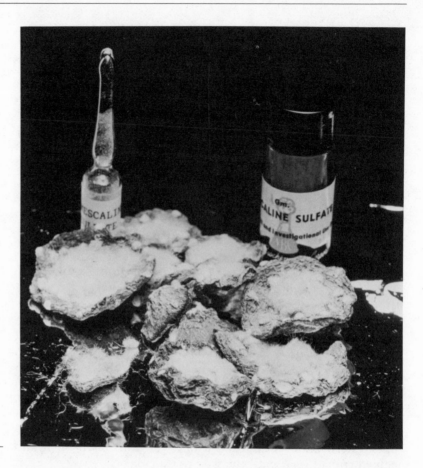

A typical dose of dried peyote "buttons," with vials of mescaline sulfate. Mescaline, the primary hallucinogenic agent in peyote, was first isolated around the turn of the century. (Jeremy Bigwood)

this way. Eventually, it won its court battles and now boasts hundreds of thousands of members throughout North America. Although Indians can use peyote legally in Native American Church ceremonies, most states prohibit non-Indians from participating.

Native American Church "meetings" begin after dark, often in tipis. The meetings take place around a fire, last all night, and include a great deal of singing, chanting, and praying, all coordinated by a leader, or "road man." Peyote is eaten throughout the night, and participants ask the spirit of the cactus to help make them better people, better able to deal with their problems. Sometimes the ritual includes elements of Christian worship. Church members tell many stories of cures of illness resulting from peyote meetings, as well as cures of alcoholism, an addiction notoriously resistant to treatment by conventional means.

Peyote has a nauseating, bitter taste that is not soon forgotten. People who try it for the first time often find it hard to swallow, and it commonly causes vomiting. After an hour or two of sickness, the discomfort usually passes. Indians say that with repeated use, especially in religious ceremonies, nausea and vomiting do not occur. A typical dose of peyote is six to twelve buttons. Some users boil them in water to make a tea, and some non-Indians even take the tea as an enema in order to avoid the bad taste and effects on the stomach.

A persistent myth in the drug subculture is that the white hairs in the centers of peyote buttons contain strychnine, which is supposed to account for the sickness. In fact, there is no strychnine in peyote (or any other hallucinogenic plant), and the hairs are just cellulose, probably indigestible but certainly not poisonous. Peyote is bitter and causes nausea because it has a lot of drugs in it — more than forty separate compounds. Chief among these is mescaline, which accounts for much of the hallucinogenic effect.

Mescaline was isolated from peyote in the late 1890s. It is the only naturally occurring psychedelic in this family of adrenaline-related drugs. Throughout the twentieth century, a few artists, philosophers, and psychologists experimented with it on themselves, but there was no general demand for it until the psychedelic revolution of the 1960s. Then black-market mescaline began to appear. However, since the drug commands a higher price than LSD, many dealers sold LSD as mescaline. Real mescaline comes as long, needlelike white crystals; half a gram is the usual dose. The pure drug may cause initial nausea, though not as frequently as peyote. Its effects last up to twelve hours and generally resemble those of the whole cactus.

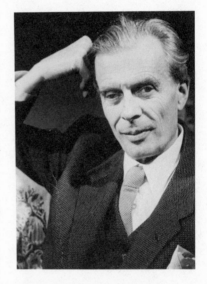

Aldous Huxley (1894–1963), the British writer and philosopher, experimented extensively with mescaline in the 1950s. (Courtesy of Laura Huxley)

STP (DOM)

STP is a synthetic drug closely resembling mescaline in its chemical structure. It produces a twelve-hour intoxication with strong stimulation and may be less euphoric than mescaline. In the late 1960s, it was blamed for an epidemic of bad trips lasting many hours. The problem was overdose; some black-market tablets contained twenty times the recommended amount. This episode left STP with such a bad reputation that few people seek it out.

MDA (Methylenedioxyamphetamine) and Related Drugs

Chemical variations of the amphetamine molecule have resulted in a number of synthetic psychedelics in this family.

MDA is the oldest and best known, first made in Germany in 1910 but not discovered to be psychoactive until much later. In doses of 100 to 150 milligrams, it produces a feeling of physical and mental well-being. In the drug subculture, MDA is known as the "love drug" because it's supposed to inspire loving feelings in groups of people. Unlike mescaline, it rarely changes visual perceptions. Although it is a strong stimulant, chemically related to amphetamine, people who take it say it calms them and promotes relaxation. Some users say it makes them more coordinated, more energetic, and better at physical activities. People often feel sluggish and drained of energy the day after taking MDA, and high doses can cause unpleasant muscular tension, especially in the face and jaw.

A newer drug, MDM (methylenedioxymethylamphetamine, also known as MDMA, Adam, and "XTC"), gives the same general effect but lasts four to six hours instead of ten to twelve. Because of its shorter duration of action, it seems gentler on the body with less day-after fatigue.

Taken by mouth in reasonable doses and in good settings, MDA and MDM rarely cause bad trips. However, these substances have gained reputations as party drugs in certain circles, with the result that some people now use them in riskier ways. Combined with alcohol or other depressants at wild parties, MDA and MDM are likelier to cause adverse reactions. Some people snort them and a few inject them intravenously; they are much more intense and dangerous by these routes. As sexual drugs, both compounds may enhance the pleasure of touching, but they interfere with erection in men and with orgasm in both men and women.

A number of other drugs exist in this series, with names like MMDA, TMA, PMA, and so on. They differ from each other in duration of action, euphoric potential, and tendency to affect visual perception. Most are pharmacological curiosities, rarely seen on the street.

Benefits and Risks of Psychedelic Drugs

Bad trips are the greatest danger of hallucinogenic drugs. Most bad trips are related to set and setting, but they also depend on dose and quality of the drug. Since legal sources of pure psychedelics do not exist, users are faced with the problem of not knowing what they are buying. All powders, pills, and capsules are suspect; only mushrooms and peyote buttons are likely to be genuine. Even good psychedelics can cause unpleasant effects if you take too much of them, and with street drugs it's not easy to determine how much is enough.

Psychedelics do not necessarily produce any particular mood or state of mind. They act as intensifiers of experience. If you take them when you are elated, they may make you superelated. If you take them when you are depressed, they may make you superdepressed. If you take them with a friend you feel totally comfortable with, they may deepen your friendship. If you take them with someone you feel uncomfortable with, they may intensify that discomfort to an unbearable degree. Therefore, if you are going to take these drugs you must be extremely careful about when, where, and with whom you take them.

Because hallucinogens are strong stimulants that make people feel very different from normal, they cannot easily be combined with everyday activity. They demand that you set time aside from ordinary routines. Possibly, their abuse potential is low just because they make this demand. Other stimulants allow people to perform ordinary activities, but it is not appropriate to take psychedelics and expect to go about your business.

Some people who take psychedelics, especially LSD, later become worried about flashbacks — brief recurrences of psychedelic symptoms that may include visual changes and "spacy" feelings. Anxiety about these experiences is more the problem than the flashbacks themselves. Actually, many people who have never taken hallucinogenic drugs also have flashbacks or experiences very much like them, which makes it seem that these are normal events in the nervous system. The best treatment for flashbacks is reassurance that nothing is seriously wrong. As people worry less about their symptoms, they pay less attention to them, and soon the flashbacks themselves fade away.

The benefits people have claimed from using psychedelics range from cures of mental and physical problems to increased appreciation of the beauty of nature to better understanding of themselves to just having good times. Some medical doctors and psychologists have been able to cure patients of serious emotional disorders by means of psychedelic therapy. There is an extensive literature on the value of using these substances occasionally and intelligently.*

You get out of the drug experience only what you put into it. The "Otherworld" from which you seek illumination is, after all, only your own psyche.
— Peter Furst, anthropologist, from his book Flesh of the Gods *(1972)*

*See the Suggested Reading at the end of this chapter.

Suggestions and Precautions for the Use of Hallucinogenic Drugs

1. Know your sources. Many fake and adulterated versions of psychedelics are sold on the street.
2. Do not attempt to pick wild psilocybin mushrooms without knowing what you are doing.
3. Cultivated psilocybin mushrooms vary greatly in potency. Get advice about dose before eating any.
4. Do not take psychedelics unless you are in good physical and psychological shape.
5. If you are trying one of the hallucinogenic drugs for the first time, take it with an experienced companion.
6. Take psychedelics only in comfortable settings on occasions when you have no responsibilities for at least the next twelve hours.
7. Remember that you may feel tired and drained of energy the following day.
8. Do not take psychedelics on a full stomach; you are less likely to feel nausea or other discomfort if your stomach is relatively empty.
9. Do not combine psychedelics with other drugs. However, the interesting effects of psychedelics sometimes wear off while their stimulation continues. If you feel agitated, restless, and unable to sleep at the end of an experience with one of these drugs, it may be appropriate to take a hypnotic dose of a sleeping pill or minor tranquilizer.
10. Remember that hallucinogenic drugs can affect perception and thinking. Do not drive, operate machinery, or engage in hazardous activities while under their influence.
11. Take psychedelics by mouth. They are more likely to cause bad reactions by other routes of administration.
12. The best experiences with these drugs result from saving them for special occasions and the right circumstances. Taking psychedelics just because they are available is less likely to produce valuable results. Taking them to get yourself out of bad moods may intensify those moods. Taking them frequently and carelessly reduces their potential to show you interesting aspects of yourself and the world around you.

Suggested Reading

Probably because they are so colorful and controversial, psychedelics are the subject of more books than most of the other categories of drugs. Many of the books are good.

Richard Evans Schultes's *Hallucinogenic Plants: A Golden Guide* (New York: Golden Press, 1976), with illustrations by Elmer W. Smith, is an inexpensive and excellent listing of all the world's psychedelic plants. In collaboration with the discoverer of LSD, Albert Hofmann, Schultes has also written *Plants of the Gods: Origins of Hallucinogenic Use* (New York: McGraw-Hill, 1979), a much larger and more beautiful work on the same subject. Another useful guide is *Hallucinogenic Plants of North America* by Jonathan Ott (Berkeley, California: Wingbow Press, 1976; revised edition, 1979).

Peter Stafford's *Psychedelics Encyclopedia* (revised edition; Los Angeles: J. P. Tarcher, 1982) covers the chemical psychedelics as well as the plants and is filled with history, description, pictures, and anecdotes.

A more comprehensive and scholarly work is *Psychedelic Drugs Reconsidered* by Lester Grinspoon and James B. Bakalar (New York: Basic Books, 1979); it contains a complete bibliography and discusses the uses of hallucinogens in psychotherapy.

Albert Hofmann reflects on his gift to the world in *LSD: My Problem Child* (New York: McGraw-Hill, 1980; translated by Jonathan Ott). With R. Gordon Wasson and Carl A. P. Ruck, he is coauthor of *The Road to Eleusis: Unveiling the Secret of the Mysteries* (New York: Harcourt Brace Jovanovich, 1978), which is a fascinating speculation on the possible use of a psychedelic potion in ancient Greek religious rites.

Two books on magic mushrooms are *Teonanácatl: Hallucinogenic Mushrooms of North America*, edited by Jonathan Ott and Jeremy Bigwood (Seattle: Madrona, 1978); and *Psilocybe Mushrooms and Their Allies* by Paul Stamets (Seattle: Homestead Book Co., 1978).

The best descriptions of the effects of yagé will be found in F. Bruce Lamb's *Wizard of the Upper Amazon: The Story of Manuel Córdova Rios* (Boston: Houghton Mifflin, 1975). The best recent work on peyote is Edward F. Anderson's *Peyote: The Divine Cactus* (Tucson: University of Arizona Press, 1980). *Shabono* by Florinda Donner (New York: Delacorte Press, 1982) is the gripping story of a young American anthropologist who lived with a South American Indian tribe; the Indians value altered states of consciousness and use a DMT snuff.

Aldous Huxley's writings on mescaline and other psychedelics are collected in *Moksha: Writings on Psychedelics and the Visionary Experience (1931–1963)*, edited by Michael Horowitz and Cynthia Palmer (New York: Stonehill, 1977). This book includes excerpts from Huxley's most famous work on the subject, his 1954 essay *The Doors of Perception* (New York: Harper & Row, 1970).

One of the few published works on MDA is Claudio Naranjo's *The Healing Journey* (New York: Ballantine Books, 1975); it discusses the author's uses of MDA and other hallucinogenic drugs in psychotherapy.

A good science-fiction novel on psychedelics is *A Time of Changes* by Robert Silverberg (New York: Signet, 1971).

So far, *Altered States* is the only movie to focus on the psychedelic experience, and it does so in a not very accurate way. *Easy Rider* and *Midnight Cowboy* have brief hallucinatory scenes.

9

Marijuana

MARIJUANA is an ancient drug, used since prehistoric times in parts of the Old World. It is a product of the hemp plant, *Cannabis sativa*, a species that also provides a useful fiber, an edible seed, an oil, and a medicine. That is a lot for one plant to do, which explains why it has always been an important cultivated crop. Cannabis is probably native to central Asia. It tends to grow in waste places around camps and settlements and has been associated with human beings for so long that it is unknown in a truly wild state.

The intoxicating properties of hemp reside in an aromatic, sticky resin exuded by the flowering tops, especially the tops of female plants. The strength of a preparation of hemp depends on the resin content; some strains produce a great deal of resin, others little. If whole plants are chopped up, leaves, stalks, and all, the resin-rich tops will be diluted by much inert material. Carefully cultivated female tops, gathered before the seeds form, are sticky to the touch with resin, highly aromatic, and very potent. The resin itself can be collected and pressed into cakes or lumps; this is hashish. Also, the resin can be extracted with solvents and concentrated into a thick, oily liquid called hash oil. Any of these preparations can be either smoked or eaten.

Marijuana is unique among the psychoactive drugs, in a class by itself. The chemicals it contains resemble no other drug

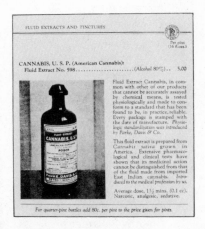

Tincture of marijuana (cannabis) was still listed in the Parke, Davis & Co. pharmaceutical catalog of 1929. (Courtesy of Tod H. Mikuriya, M.D.)

molecules. Unlike most of the substances discussed in this book, they are insoluble in water but very soluble in oil. Therefore, they are absorbed unevenly when eaten, and they stay in the body for a long time because they accumulate in body fat. Marijuana is neither a stimulant nor a depressant, but has some features of both. Many people regard it as a mild psychedelic, but its effects are different from those of the true hallucinogens, and it is not necessarily mild. Moreover, the abuse potential of marijuana is considerably higher than that of psychedelics, because it can be used frequently or continually in combination with everyday activities.

As a psychoactive drug, cannabis has a much longer history in other parts of the world than it does in Western countries. Europeans and Americans grew the plant exclusively for its fiber for many years, and even when tincture of cannabis was widely used in Western medicine in the 1800s, few people took it to get high or reported that they felt high when they did take it. The knowledge of how to smoke hemp was probably brought to Brazil by black slaves who used the plant in Africa; the practice traveled north to Mexico and, finally, reached the United States.

Marijuana smoking began in the United States after World War I. Introduced by Mexican migrant workers, it caught on first among black people in southern cities. Many of its early users were musicians. Over the years, it spread to other subgroups, but was rarely associated with the white middle class

Marijuana growing on the United States government's experimental farm at the University of Mississippi. (Timothy Plowman)

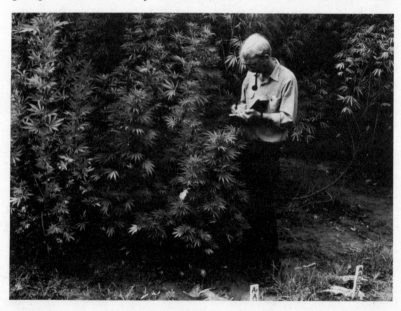

until the 1960s, when it became a prominent symbol of the youth movement on college campuses. Since then, it has grown steadily more popular and today is the most widely used of all the illegal drugs.

From the very first, marijuana — which is known by many slang names, including pot, grass, and smoke — provoked a great deal of contention, mostly as a result of its associations. It was the drug of deviant subcultures and minority races even before it got mixed up with hippies and revolutionaries. Despite its growing acceptance today, the dominant culture still views it as a dangerous drug, worse than alcohol and tobacco, likely to lead to heroin.

In this highly charged atmosphere, arguments about marijuana tend to be more political than factual. And because pharmacologists and medical doctors are just as caught up in the politics of marijuana as other people, it's difficult to get neutral information about the drug. Much marijuana research sets out to prove preconceived ideas, and much of it is not worth reading.

Politics aside, the effects of marijuana are hard to describe, because they are so variable — more so than those of other drugs. Some of this variation has to do with set and setting, but some is inherent in the drug.

People who smoke marijuana for the first time often feel nothing at all, even if they take high doses of strong pot. As with other psychoactive substances, people have to learn to associate changes of consciousness with the physical effects of the drug. Compared to other drugs, however, the physical effects of marijuana are not spectacular. It makes the heart beat somewhat faster, causes the mouth and eyes to become dry, and reddens the whites of the eyes. Of these, the most noticeable change is the dryness of the mouth. Only people who wear contact lenses are likely to notice the dryness of the eyes. Increased heart rate is easily ignored, although it can become the basis of a panic reaction in anxious first-time users, who may interpret it to mean they are having heart attacks.

When people learn to get high on marijuana, their early experiences with it are often quite lively. Everything may strike them funny, and all sensory experiences become novel and interesting. Listening to music, eating, and making love can become more than usually absorbing. Time seems long and drawn out. People sometimes have strange illusions, such as seeing a room expand or feeling as though their legs have become enormously long.

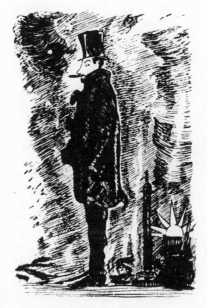

Charles Baudelaire (1821–1867): a self-portrait by the French poet from 1844, drawn under the influence of hashish. (Fitz Hugh Ludlow Memorial Library)

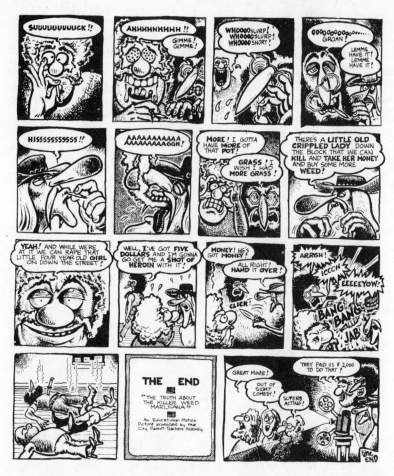

(From *The Further Adventures of the Fabulous Furry Freak Brothers* by Gilbert Shelton. Copyright © 1979 Rip Off Press, Inc.)

With repeated use, these remarkable effects tend to fade away. Regular users may find that pot makes them relaxed or more sociable without greatly affecting their perceptions or moods. Very heavy users usually feel little from the drug, often smoking it simply out of habit.

Bad reactions to marijuana are more likely when high doses of strong material are taken in bad settings, especially by inexperienced users. Most are simple panic reactions, easily treated with reassurance that everything will be all right as soon as the drug wears off. The effects of smoking marijuana usually diminish after an hour and disappear after two or three hours. Some people, if they have smoked a lot of pot, feel tired or "fuzzy" the next morning.

Some users find that marijuana stimulates them and keeps them awake at night; others use it to help them fall asleep. It makes some people depressed and irritable, and others groggy for several hours. Possibly, some kinds of pot are more sedative than others. In recent years, stronger and stronger marijuana has become available. Some of the very potent sinsemilla ("without seed") from California is as potent as hashish and can be disorienting to people who are not used to it.

Taken by mouth, rather than smoked, marijuana is a stronger drug, slower to come on, with longer-lasting effects. Because the resin is insoluble in water, marijuana tea is not very effective. But the crude drug can be added to food, and the active principles are easily extracted in alcohol or fat. Although some users like to eat cannabis, most prefer to smoke it because it's less trouble, and the effect comes on very fast. The main problem with oral use is the risk of overdosage. Since the stomach absorbs the drug unevenly, the right dosage is hard to estimate, and it's easy to take too much. Overdoses of cannabis are unpleasant, though not dangerous. They can make people extremely disoriented and delirious, as if suffering from a high fever, and are often followed by stupor and hangover. Perhaps because oral use requires more preparation and produces stronger effects, people who eat marijuana are less likely to become dependent on it than people who smoke it.

Whether they eat it or smoke it, users frequently combine marijuana with other drugs, such as alcohol, downers, stimulants, and even psychedelics. The effects of these combinations are not predictable, depending more on the individual than on the drugs. Because marijuana is not as powerful or as toxic as most of the other drugs, there is no special pharmacological danger in mixing it (as there is, say, in mixing alcohol with downers). Still, users should be aware that combinations they are not used to may disagree with them and may produce unexpectedly strong effects.

The medical safety of marijuana is great. It does not kill people in overdose or produce other symptoms of obvious toxicity. Used occasionally, it is no more of a health problem than the occasional use of coffee or tea, and certainly it is less toxic than alcohol and tobacco.

Long-term, regular marijuana smoking can, however, significantly irritate the respiratory tract, causing chronic, dry coughs that resemble the coughs of some cigarette smokers. Further, marijuana smoke may contain more tars than tobacco smoke, and can probably produce lung and bronchial disease in susceptible individuals. The risk depends on how much users smoke over how long a time.

Aside from respiratory irritation, heavy marijuana use does not seem to cause other medical problems. Of course, warnings of the medical dangers of cannabis have been well publicized, with reports of everything from brain damage to injury of the immune and reproductive systems, but these are based on poor research, often conducted by passionate foes of the drug. Studies of populations that have smoked cannabis for many years do not reveal obvious illnesses that can be linked to marijuana.

Much has been made of the fact that tetrahydrocannabinol, or THC, the most active chemical in cannabis resin, accumulates in body fat, staying around for weeks after the last dose of marijuana is smoked. Although this is true, and it is very different from the pattern of quick elimination of water-soluble drugs, it is not a problem in itself. If THC were a very toxic drug, its persistence in body fat would be cause for concern, but THC and marijuana are less toxic than most of the drugs discussed in this book.*

Psychological problems related to regular use of marijuana are also subjects of controversy. Opponents of the drug charge that it interferes with memory and intellectual functioning and leads to an amotivational syndrome in which people lose their initiative and will to work. There is no question that young people who lack motivation often smoke a lot of pot and do very little else, but it is doubtful that marijuana made them that way. Heavy pot smoking is more likely to be a symptom of amotivation than a cause of it, and those same young people would probably be wasting their time in other ways or with other drugs if pot were not available.

I started dealing dope 'cause it was the only way I could afford to buy dope. Now I do it for the money.
— *sixteen-year-old boy*

---

*Marijuana may be quite toxic if it is contaminated with paraquat, a very poisonous chemical herbicide used to kill unwanted plants. In 1975 American drug enforcement authorities began encouraging officials in Mexico to spray this poison from helicopters on the illegal marijuana fields of that country. The growers soon learned that if they harvested their pot immediately after it was sprayed, it would still look healthy and could be sold to dealers as usual. In this way, paraquat-contaminated Mexican marijuana began to find its way to users in the United States.

The exact dangers of smoking paraquat are unclear, but it is certain that it cannot be good for you; the only question is how bad it is. Apparently it can cause serious lung damage over time and may affect other organs as well. There is no easy way to spot paraquat on a sample of pot, but some drug testing labs can analyze for it. Although public outcry put an end to American support for the Mexican program, the drug enforcement authorities are again pressing for use of paraquat on marijuana fields, both in other countries and in the major producing states, such as California and Florida. If they have their way, paraquat contamination will again be a risk to all users who do not grow their own pot or know who grew it. Some thoughtful legislators have urged that paraquat be mixed with some distinctive odor or color that would warn users of contaminated material, but so far that is just a suggestion.

As for its effects on memory and intellect, heavy users sometimes say that marijuana makes their minds fuzzy and can interfere with memory. These effects seem to disappear when people cut down on their use of the drug or stop using it altogether.

Although dependence on marijuana certainly occurs and has become more common as use of the drug has increased, it does not exactly resemble dependence on any other psychoactive drug. At its worst, marijuana dependence consists of chain smoking, from the moment of getting up in the morning to the time of falling asleep — a pattern similar to that of many cigarette smokers. But dramatic withdrawal syndromes don't occur when people suddenly stop using marijuana, and craving for the drug is not nearly as intense as for tobacco, alcohol, or narcotics.

Tolerance to marijuana also occurs. Even the strongest varieties seem to lose their power if people smoke them day in and day out. This leads heavy users to keep searching for more potent pot so they can feel stoned again. In fact, all they really need to do is cut back on their frequency of use; even a twenty-four-hour break from the routine of smoking all day long will allow a heavy user to become sensitive again to the psychoactive properties of marijuana.

Although dependence on marijuana has fewer physical components than dependence on more toxic drugs, it can still be very hard to break and very upsetting to people who find themselves caught up in it. Some heavy users are unable to stop smoking even though they no longer get useful effects from pot and, in fact, get effects they actively dislike, such as strong sedation and chronic coughs. Recently, self-help groups modeled on Alcoholics Anonymous have sprung up for people with unwanted marijuana habits.

Marijuana dependence can be sneaky in its development. It doesn't appear overnight like cigarette addiction, or in a matter of weeks like heroin addiction, but rather builds up over a long time. In most cases, people begin smoking pot only in special, usually social, situations. At first, because the drug causes such strong effects, they cannot imagine smoking it at other times. With increasing use, however, tolerance develops, and also people learn to adapt to being high. Soon they can perform normal activities while under the influence of marijuana. Users may then begin to smoke during the day, perhaps by themselves. With time, and unless precautions are taken, marijuana smoke can gradually pervade all their waking hours. At that point, the habit is not easy to break.

Eventually I became a daily pot smoker, sometimes starting in the morning. It was my main way of relating to other people. However, I started getting less and less effect from it that I liked. In fact, it began to make me groggy and sleepy most of the time and also gave me a cough. These unwelcome effects got worse and worse until I realized I would have to stop using pot. So I made a resolution to quit completely.

Well, it surprised me to find that wasn't so easy. It took me three years of trying before I really gave up smoking marijuana, even though I no longer got pleasant effects from it. I never realized how much of a habit I had and how hooked I was on it . . .
— forty-one-year-old man, lawyer

Even in heaviest usage marijuana does not lead to heroin or any other drug. Many junkies smoked marijuana before they tried opiates, but few marijuana users take narcotics. Many junkies also drank alcohol heavily before they discovered heroin, sometimes at very young ages, yet no one argues that alcohol leads to heroin. The reason, of course, is that alcohol enjoys general social approval, while marijuana is a "bad" drug and so invites false attributions of causality. Possibly, marijuana users are more likely than nonusers to try psychedelics and cocaine, because the distribution networks of these drugs overlap somewhat, but there is no quality of marijuana that induces its users to become consumers of other substances.

Adaptation to marijuana enables users to learn to perform well under its influence. Unlike alcohol, it does not invariably depress reflexes and reaction times. People who aren't used to its effects will not be able to drive cars well or do any number of other routine tasks well while stoned. Even experienced users need time to practice a given task under the influence of marijuana in order to bring performance up to normal. Some users feel that marijuana helps them concentrate and enables them to work better, but even they have to learn to adapt to its effects. Most scientific tests show that marijuana impairs performance of all sorts. It is easy to come up with such results if you give marijuana to people who are not used to it, give it in much higher doses than they are used to, or give them hard tasks to perform, especially tasks they have never done while stoned.

Many marijuana smokers drive cars, fly airplanes, ski, scuba dive, and engage in other hazardous activities after smoking. Many of them get away with it because they are experienced users with practice. This does not change the fact that marijuana can drastically interfere with performance in some circumstances. Pot and driving may not be as bad a combination for everyone as drinking and driving, but it is certainly not a good one. For teen-agers who drive recklessly to begin with, it can be especially dangerous.

Devotees of marijuana like to argue its merits, trying to persuade others that it is really a beneficial drug. In fact, cannabis was used in medicine in the past, and some doctors today feel that it is still a valuable remedy for some ailments. Current federal laws prohibit all uses of marijuana, but synthetic THC is available for research, and many states have now legalized marijuana for specific therapeutic uses.

Both THC and marijuana are good treatments for nausea and vomiting. Doctors have used them successfully with cancer

I have multiple sclerosis. About three years after it was diagnosed I discovered marijuana. A friend told me it was relaxing. My main problem then, aside from partial blindness, was tenseness and tremors in my muscles. Pot cured it, and I've smoked regularly ever since, about four to five times a week. If I go without it for a week, the muscle tremors come back . . . Most people with MS have repeated attacks and keep losing body function. I'm convinced that pot has kept me in remission all these years.
— forty-one-year-old man, part-time roofer

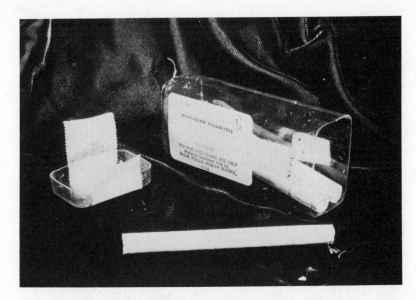

Government-manufactured marijuana cigarettes. A few patients with glaucoma have been able to obtain them legally for the treatment of that eye disease. (Jeremy Bigwood)

patients receiving chemotherapy, which involves very toxic drugs that often cause intense stomach upsets. This effect was first discovered by teen-agers with leukemia who happened to be pot heads. Cannabis may also help asthma patients breathe easier, but not in the form of joints because the smoke may make them cough. It also is a specific treatment for glaucoma, a serious eye disease in which fluid pressure builds up in the eyeball, causing losses of vision. Marijuana reduces this pressure. Finally, it relaxes stiff muscles in a condition called spastic paralysis that results from brain injuries and diseases such as multiple sclerosis.

Although many patients prefer the effect of marijuana to that of pure THC, federal agencies won't permit doctors to prescribe the natural plant. Yet THC is not the same as whole marijuana and may not be as safe. Recently, several pharmaceutical companies have come up with synthetic drugs related to THC and have tried to market them as antinausea remedies. In general, they are much more toxic than marijuana.

Aside from these specific uses, many people find that pot relieves the symptoms of various mild ailments, from headaches to menstrual cramps. Probably, they use the marijuana to get high and use the high as a way of taking their minds off discomfort. Sometimes taking your attention away from the symptoms of a minor ailment will allow it to subside. The less frequently you smoke marijuana, the more likely it is to work for you as a medicine.

Of course, the same principle applies to getting high from pot. The less frequently you use it, the better and more intense will be your experiences with it. The main danger of smoking marijuana is simply that it will get away from you, becoming more and more of a repetitive habit and less and less of a useful way of changing consciousness. The ease of integrating marijuana smoking with all activities, from parties to sports to watching television, favors habitual use. Also, tolerance to the interesting effects of the drug often encourages users to smoke more of it, when in fact they should be cutting down to increase their sensitivity. The absence of dramatic negative effects, such as hangovers, further encourages overuse. Unless you set rules for when and where you will smoke, you are likely to find yourself using pot more than you should — to the point where all the interesting and useful effects of the drug disappear and you are left with a stubborn, unproductive habit.

Some Suggestions for Using Marijuana Wisely

1. Define what benefits you want from pot. Do not use it just because other people do or because it is available. Be aware of the dangers associated with acquiring an illegal drug.*

2. If you get effects you like from marijuana, you will have to take precautions if you want to keep enjoying them.

3. Set limits on usage. For example, you may want to use pot only with certain friends, only on weekends, or only when you have no work to do. Such rules are necessary if you want to prevent your use from turning into a habit that gives you little satisfaction.

4. Remember that it can be dangerous to drive, operate machinery, or engage in hazardous activities under the influence of marijuana. The drug can cause illusions of time and space and always takes getting used to.

5. If you find the effects you like from marijuana becoming less intense or disappearing altogether, *stop using it*. You can resume after a break and get them back. The trick is to keep frequency of use below the level where you become insensitive to marijuana's interesting effects on consciousness. Odd as it may sound, less is more, and you can easily prove that to yourself.

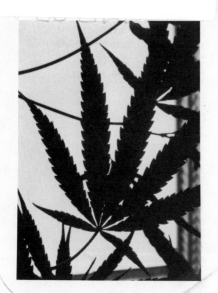

(Michael R. Aldrich)

*See pages 163–67.

6. If you find that the effects you like are disappearing, the worst things you can do are smoke more or look for stronger pot. Those actions will just increase the problem.

7. Consider using marijuana by eating it in some form rather than smoking it. It is more trouble to take by mouth and the effects are different, but the risk of dependence is less.

8. Be careful about combining marijuana with other psychoactive drugs.

9. Be careful about set and setting, especially if trying marijuana for the first time.

10. Do not use marijuana on the job or at school. Most people would not drink alcohol in those situations, and just because pot is less detectable is no reason to use it. The more situations in which you allow yourself to smoke, the more likely you are to become dependent.

11. If you develop a cough or wheeze, or become more susceptible to chest colds, marijuana may be doing harm to your respiratory tract. Stop using it, cut down on use, or switch to eating it.

12. If you find that you are using marijuana more than you want and are not getting useful effects from it, consider the possibility that it is controlling you more than you are controlling it. Try to do without it for a while. If you cannot, you may need outside help in breaking the habit.

Suggested Reading

Much has been published about marijuana in recent years, but few books worth reading exist.

The best general history of marijuana is *Marihuana: The First Twelve Thousand Years* by Ernest L. Abel (London: Plenum Press, 1980). *Marijuana Botany* by Robert Connell Clarke (Berkeley, California: And/Or Press, 1981) is about the plant itself. It is lavishly illustrated.

The Marijuana Papers, edited by David Solomon (New York: Bobbs-Merrill, 1966), is an anthology of historical, literary, sociological, and medical articles that is still valuable reading. *Marihuana Reconsidered* by Lester Grinspoon (Cambridge, Massachusetts: Harvard University Press, 1971) is a comprehensive overview of the drug by a psychiatrist. The origins and development of marijuana prohibition in America are discussed in Richard J. Bonnie and Charles H. Whitebread's *Marihuana Conviction: A History of Marihuana Prohibition in the United States* (Charlottesville, Virginia: University Press of Virginia, 1974).

One of the most readable and informative books on effects and uses of pot is *High Culture: Marijuana in the Lives of Americans* by William Novak (New York: Knopf, 1980). One example of a crusading antimarijuana book is *Keep Off the Grass* by Gabriel G. Nahas (New York: Pergamon Press, 1979). One example of a promarijuana book, written for users, is *A Child's Garden of Grass* by Jack S. Margolis and Richard Clorfene (New York: Ballantine, 1978).

Louisa May Alcott wrote a short story about hashish in 1865. Titled "Perilous Play," it is reprinted in *Plots and Counterplots: More Unknown Thrillers of Louisa May Alcott*, edited by Madeleine Stern (New York: William Morrow, 1976). A modern comic novel filled with references to marijuana is *The Fan Man* by William Kotzwinkle (New York: Avon Books, 1974). Its hero, a delightful character named Horse Badorties, is never without pot.

Although teen-agers make up the bulk of the movie-going public, few films have capitalized on the popularity of marijuana among young people. Three notable exceptions are *Up in Smoke* and *Nice Dreams* with Cheech and Chong, and Peter Fonda's classic from the 1960s, *Easy Rider*. An outrageous antimarijuana propaganda film from the 1930s, *Reefer Madness*, now plays on college campuses and in "art" movie houses, usually to the delight of mostly stoned audiences.

10

Solvents and Inhalants; Deliriants; PCP and Ketamine

T HE DRUGS DESCRIBED in this chapter are a strange assortment of chemicals and plants that do not fit neatly into other categories. Some of them are more toxic than the substances discussed earlier, and, though all of them have their devoted fans, experienced users regard them as second-rate or substitute drugs, not worth taking unless preferred drugs are unavailable.

Organic Solvents

In chemistry the word *organic* refers to compounds of carbon. Some of the simplest organic chemicals are clear, volatile liquids made by distilling petroleum. These liquids have many uses in industry. Some, like gasoline, make good fuels because they burn readily. Others, like benzene and toluene, dissolve grease and oil, making them useful as cleaning fluids and solvents.

The fumes of these organic solvents have strong chemical odors and make people feel lightheaded, hot, and dizzy. Cans and bottles of them usually carry warning labels about using them only with good ventilation. Many people dislike breathing solvent fumes, but some find it interesting and repeatedly sniff certain household products or gasoline to change their state of consciousness. Products containing organic solvents include some glues (rubber cement and model airplane glue); paint thinner; lighter fluid; and varnish, wax, and spot removers.

As psychoactive drugs, the organic solvents produce effects resembling low doses of general anesthetics, but they are more toxic and tend to cause dizziness, nausea, and other uncomfortable physical feelings. In high doses they may induce visual hallucinations and vivid waking dreams. Some young people find that the effects are similar to the dizzy excitement that comes from spinning around. Since many children use spinning as a technique for changing awareness, and since organic solvents are commonly found around the house, many children come to experiment with them. Often these chemicals are a child's first introduction to consciousness-change by means of drugs.

Children who regularly sniff solvents develop tolerance to them. Although there is no physical withdrawal as with alcohol and narcotics, the sniffing habit can be very difficult to break. Just like grown-up drunks, solvent-sniffing children may spend most of their waking time in stupors, unable to do their work or pay attention to what really matters.

Probably some people have sniffed solvents occasionally over the years just as some people have played with chloroform, ether, and nitrous oxide. For the most part, this use never attracted much notice. Beginning about 1959, however, newspapers in the United States began to focus attention on glue-sniffing as a new drug menace spreading among children in cities of the West and Midwest. A few children died from lack of oxygen by putting glue in plastic bags, then putting the bags over their heads. Seizing upon these cases, newspapers dramatized the hazards of glue-sniffing, making it seem extremely dangerous. Parents' groups and police officials then called for laws against it. The main effect of all this attention was to stimulate curiosity about glue-sniffing and cause a tremendous increase in the numbers of people doing it. At the beginning of the 1960s, gasoline sniffing was the most popular form of organic solvent use. Sniffing of other substances was rare and caused no concern. Then came a hysterical nationwide crusade against glue-sniffing with scare stories in newspapers, legislative hearings, and finally, arrest and imprisonment of some children. Only glue-sniffing received this kind of attention, and only glue-sniffing became enormously popular. Today, significant numbers of schoolchildren have tried or used glue in attempts to get high.

TAJAR: What made you want to smell gas, Bullet?
BULLET: Well, when you feel bad, you smell it and it makes you feel kind of hot and kind of drowsy, like you was floating through the air. It makes you feel sort of hot inside and different from the way you were before . . .
TAJAR: Bullet, how come so much gas was spilled on the cellar floor?
BULLET: Oh, I just wanted to get more on my rag. If you have a lot it makes you sort of dream. It gets all dark and you see shooting stars in it, and this time I saw big flies flying in it. They were big and green and had white wings.
— from an interview with a young gasoline sniffer, in Licit and Illicit Drugs, *by Edward M. Brecher and the editors of* Consumer Reports *(1972)*

All of the scare stories exaggerated the dangers of solvent inhalation, saying that it certainly led to brain, heart, and liver damage, destruction of the bone marrow, blindness, and death. There *is* medical evidence of harm from exposure to organic solvents, but most of it concerns factory workers who breathe the fumes all day long over months and years or rare individuals who drink the liquids. Young people who sniff solvents occasionally are not likely to develop serious medical problems.

As with alcohol, anesthetics, and the other depressants, use of solvents can produce disorientation and impairment of judgment and coordination. Since these changes favor accidents, it is silly to sniff solvent fumes while driving or doing anything else requiring good reflexes. Overdoses of fumes may lead to unconsciousness, and with complete lack of oxygen, death is a real possibility. Also, it may be unwise to mix sniffing with drinking, both because that combination puts a great deal of stress on the liver and because it can depress respiration to a dangerous degree. In pregnant women, solvent fumes may raise the risk of birth defects. Fumes of some of the solvents can irritate the membranes of the nose.

Inhalation puts these chemicals into the blood and brain very fast, so the effects come on almost immediately. They usually last from fifteen minutes to half an hour after sniffing stops. Some people breathe fumes directly from containers; others put solvents or glue on rags or in paper bags.

The majority of sniffers are between the ages of ten and seventeen, with children of certain ethnic groups predominating. The most common sniffers have been Hispanic males. Many Native American boys also sniff solvents — a source of great concern on many Indian reservations. Black children, on the other hand, seem to prefer other drugs, and until recently, few girls used solvents. No one knows why these differences exist, and today, with rising use of all drugs among young people, the older patterns may be changing.

Grownups tend to regard glue, gasoline, paint thinner, and the rest as cheap highs — easy to obtain and not very good. Among people who have tried many drugs, the organic solvents are always considered low-class and second-rate, much inferior to drugs such as alcohol and marijuana. The popularity of solvents among children reflects their easy availability and dramatic power to change consciousness fast rather than any really desirable qualities about them. When children grow up and discover other drugs that are less toxic and more useful, they generally stop playing around with solvents.

Aerosol Propellants

Aerosol spray cans are pressurized with other organic chemicals. Until recently, most aerosol products contained types of fluorocarbons known by the brand name Freon. Freon, when inhaled, produces the same effects as the organic solvents and presents the same risks to the user. Because of increasing concern of scientists that so much Freon being sprayed into the air might do permanent harm to the earth's atmosphere, some manufacturers have switched to other propellants, usually simpler organic compounds that also cause changes in consciousness when people inhale them.

Inhaling aerosol propellants is a bit more complicated than inhaling solvents because the propellants come mixed with other substances. For example, when you press the button on a can of black spray paint, what comes out is a cloud of tiny droplets of black paint and Freon gas. Inhaling black paint does not get you high and can make you very sick. Some users solve this problem by spraying the can into a bag or balloon so that the particles separate from the Freon gas by adhering to the sides. Others turn the cans upside down so that only Freon comes out, and still others inhale the sprays through cloth filters.

Nitrite Inhalants

Amyl Nitrite (Amys, Poppers, Snappers, Pearls, Aspirol, Vaporal)

Amyl nitrite is a simple chemical that has been used for more than a hundred years to relieve heart pain in people who suffer from coronary artery disease. Such people often feel severe chest pain when they exert themselves. If they breathe the fumes of amyl nitrite, the pain quickly disappears because the drug dilates arteries throughout the body, reducing the workload of the heart. Other effects are a sudden fall in blood pressure, a throbbing feeling in the head (or even a brief, pounding headache), occasional dizziness and nausea, warmth and flushing of the skin, and a dramatically altered state of consciousness that reminds some people of fainting or going under general anesthesia.

Amyl nitrite is a clear, yellowish liquid with a strong chemical smell. It comes in inhalers and in cloth-covered glass capsules that can be crushed in the hand and sniffed. (They break with an audible "pop" — hence the common street name *poppers*.) Until 1960, amyl nitrite was a prescription drug. Although some people used it recreationally, most buyers were heart patients who carried it with them for medical purposes and did not think of it as a mind-changing substance. Then the Food and Drug Administration removed the prescription requirement, so that amyl nitrite became an over-the-counter drug, available to anyone.

During the 1960s, many users of street drugs experimented with amyl nitrite as a quick, legal high. It appealed especially to young people, to those who liked to sniff organic solvents, and to those who liked the highs of general anesthetics. In addition, poppers had a special reputation as enhancers of sexual experience. Inhaled during a sexual act, the drug is supposed to intensify the experience and prolong and intensify orgasm. Although some heterosexual men and women use it in this way, male homosexuals have been the greatest fans of amyl nitrite. The effects of a single, deep inhalation last only for a few minutes and are often followed by less pleasant sensations, but gay men may pass the drug back and forth many times while having sex.

As recreational use of amyl nitrite spread, authorities opposed its unrestricted sale. Finally, in 1969, the Food and Drug Administration reimposed the prescription requirement, ending over-the-counter distribution. Today, however, it is still in wide use, especially in gay communities.

All nitrites are poisonous in excess, but amyl nitrite, when inhaled, breaks down easily and leaves the body very quickly. It is considered one of the safest drugs in medicine, and even people who inhale it frequently do not seem to suffer ill effects. Still, it is probably not wise to overdo it. The strong chemical odor of amyl nitrite is suggestive of materials that are hard on the body; it is possible that long-term use has physical consequences doctors do not yet recognize. It should not be used at all by people with anemia, glaucoma, high blood pressure, or recent head injuries. Also, it may be harmful to pregnant women. Because the liquid drug can corrode the cornea, users should be careful to keep it away from their eyes.

Because amyl nitrite causes a sudden drop in blood pressure, it can produce loss of coordination and fainting. It should not be inhaled in situations requiring muscular coordination or careful posture. Also, it should be used with good ventilation and never be put into closed containers, such as plastic bags, for continuous breathing. As with organic solvents, that method can lead to suffocation.

I was first introduced to amyl nitrite during my senior year in college. The father of one of my friends had a heart condition for which he used the drug. He would amass huge numbers of poppers and give them out to anyone who wanted them . . . The effect was immediate. My arms and legs felt like liquid warmth, and at the same time I got a pounding in my head . . . When I exhaled, my vision blurred, with small blue patches filling my field of vision . . .
— twenty-year-old man, medical student

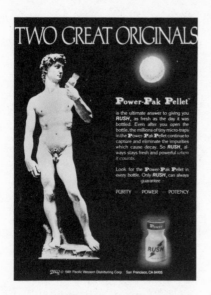

(Courtesy of Pacific Western
Distributing Corp.)

Butyl Nitrite and Isobutyl Nitrite (Locker Room, Rush)

Butyl nitrite and isobutyl nitrite are close chemical relatives of
amyl nitrite that are not under any drug regulations. They are
sold by mail order and over the counter in head shops. They
come in small bottles or aerosol cans with labels identifying
them as "liquid incense" or "room odorizer," but everyone who
buys these products knows what they are for. Butyl nitrite and
isobutyl nitrite are of recent appearance as recreational drugs.
Their effects are the same as those of poppers.

Some Precautions About Organic Solvents and Inhalants

1. Organic solvents are highly flammable. Never use them
    near open flames or sparks.
2. People have died of asphyxiation by putting their heads in
    plastic bags containing small amounts of solvents.
3. Never sniff solvents while driving, operating machinery, or
    engaging in other hazardous activities requiring good
    reflexes, coordination, and attention.
4. If you sniff solvents, get plenty of fresh air afterward to
    flush the chemical out of your system.
5. Do not sniff solvents while drinking alcohol or using other
    depressants.
6. Do not sniff solvents if you have a history of liver disease.
7. Regular sniffing of solvents can become a stubborn drug
    habit, much like alcoholism. If you develop this pattern of
    use, you may need outside help to break it.
8. Remember that people who are most experienced with
    psychoactive drugs always say that organic solvents are
    second-rate.
9. Amyl, butyl, and isobutyl nitrite are less toxic than organic
    solvents and not as flammable. They should be used only
    with good ventilation and not breathed continuously.
10. Only inhale nitrites when you are in a comfortable sitting
    or lying position.
11. Be careful not to get liquid nitrites in your eyes.

Deliriants

Delirium is a state of mental disturbance marked by confusion
and disorientation. People in delirium cannot think clearly and

may not remember who they are, where they are, or what year it is. They may also hallucinate, seeing and hearing things that are not there. Usually, delirium is a temporary condition resulting from some disorder of the brain. For example, a high fever will cause delirium; when the fever comes down, the delirium ends. If you can remember the experience of a high fever as a young child, you know what delirium is.

Most psychoactive drugs will cause delirium in overdoses by being temporarily toxic to the brain. This kind of delirium is called a toxic psychosis because it is a malfunction of the brain owing to the presence of a toxin in the body. As the drug overdose is metabolized and eliminated, the toxic psychosis resolves. If delirium is very strong, people may not remember it clearly afterward; that is, they may have some degree of amnesia for the experience.

Depending on what causes the delirium, there may be physical effects as well, usually uncomfortable ones such as nausea, dizziness, headache, and prostration. The mental experiences are variable, too, and although many people find them unpleasant, some find them powerfully fascinating, more vivid than ordinary reality. Here is one man's description of a visual hallucination he had as a child during a high fever:

"I was standing on a cliff looking down at an ocean of cream. Somehow I knew that the cream was just about to curdle, and there was something absolutely horrible about that. But the tension just kept building and building. The ocean of cream was always just on the point of curdling, and the tension was unbearable. It is one of the most vivid memories of my childhood."

Some drugs, called deliriants, cause delirium at subtoxic doses. They are a strange group of plants and chemicals derived from them. Some of them have been used for thousands of years to induce altered states of consciousness. They certainly do not appeal to all people, and some of them are dangerous. Nevertheless, they remain popular.

Nightshades (Jimsonweed, Datura, Belladonna, Henbane)

The nightshade family of plants includes some very popular foods: tomatoes, sweet and hot peppers, eggplants, and potatoes. It also includes tobacco and some poisonous plants that are infamous because of their associations with crime, witchcraft, and black magic. Even their names are sinister: henbane, mandrake, and deadly nightshade, for example. Nightshades look scary, too. They are rank, hairy plants with strange smells and peculiar flowers; some have dangerous fruit.

In North America the main poisonous nightshades are two species of datura: *Datura stramonium*, or jimsonweed, in the East and *Datura meteloides*, or sacred datura, in the West. Sacred datura is so called because of its long involvement with Native American magic and religion.

All parts of these plants contain scopolamine, a drug that causes delirium and can be seriously poisonous in high doses. The lowest concentration of scopolamine is in the roots, making them the safest parts of the plant. Highest concentrations are in the seeds, making them the most dangerous. Roots, seeds, leaves, and flowers can all be eaten, smoked, brewed into teas, or even ground up in fat and rubbed on the skin. All of these methods put scopolamine into the bloodstream and cause intoxication.

The physical effects of scopolamine are very dramatic and often very uncomfortable. They include parched mouth and burning thirst; hot, dry skin and a feverish feeling; widely dilated eyes (making bright light painful); inability to focus the eyes at close distances; rapid heart rate; constipation; difficulty in urinating; and, in men, interference with ejaculation. These effects may last for twelve to forty-eight hours after a single dose of datura.

The mental effects are equally dramatic: restlessness, disorientation, and other symptoms of delirium, including vivid hallucinations that may seem so real that people lose all contact with ordinary reality. Because scopolamine usually leaves you with some amnesia, it is often hard to remember these hallucinations clearly when the drug wears off. Going into other worlds is fascinating, but the worlds datura takes people to can be frightening, populated by monsters and devils and filled with violent, frenzied energy.

The ability of plants containing scopolamine to disconnect people from ordinary reality accounts for their popularity in certain circles. Criminals have used them for centuries in all parts of the world, slipping them to unsuspecting victims to make it easier to rob, rape, or kidnap them. Witches in medieval Europe used deadly nightshade (belladonna), henbane, and mandrake to have the experience of flying and to meet the Devil in their visions. American Indian medicine men have used jimsonweed and sacred datura to initiate young men into the mysteries of the spirit world and to seek visions in group religious rituals.

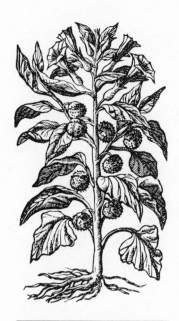

Datura stramonium: jimsonweed, or thornapple, as pictured in an herbal from 1636. (Fitz Hugh Ludlow Memorial Library)

Today datura seems to appeal mostly to young people seeking strong intoxication. The plant is easily available in many places and is very powerful. It is in wide use as a recreational drug, often in combination with alcohol, among teen-agers on Indian reservations in the West. Drug crisis centers throughout the United States see frequent cases of bad trips on datura.

Although medical doctors consider datura very dangerous, it will probably not do physical harm to the average healthy person. The main danger of datura is accidental death or injury resulting from disorientation. For example, people intoxicated on this plant have drowned by stumbling into deep bodies of water, possibly in an effort to quench the thirst and fever caused by scopolamine. Others, experiencing monsters chasing them, have taken serious falls.

Scopolamine is still used as a medical drug. Until recently, low doses of it went into over-the-counter sleeping pills, and some cold and allergy tablets still include it to dry up runny noses. Higher doses are occasionally given by injection to women in labor ("Twilight Sleep") to make them amnesic for the experience of childbirth, a practice that does not seem beneficial to either mother or baby because it produces a predictable violent delirium. Jimsonweed leaves have been rolled into cigarettes for the treatment of asthma, and tincture of belladonna is still used to treat gastrointestinal spasms.

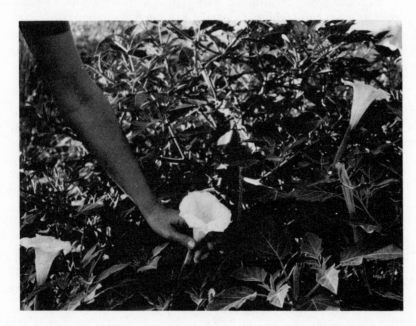

Sacred datura, *Datura meteloides*, growing along a roadside near Tucson, Arizona. (Andrew Weil)

Amanita Mushrooms (Fly Agaric, *Amanita muscaria;* Panther Mushroom, *Amanita pantherina)*

Amanitas are a family of large, beautiful mushrooms that grow in many parts of the world. Some of them are deadly, the most poisonous of all wild mushrooms. Some are edible and delicious. Two are neither deadly nor edible as food but are used as psychoactive drugs.

Amanita muscaria, or the fly agaric, is the big mushroom with white dots on a red or orange cap. (*Agaric* is an old word for mushroom; the name *fly* comes from an old practice of chopping this mushroom into a saucer of milk to attract and kill flies.) The fly agaric is often pictured in illustrations of fairy tales and cannot be mistaken for any other mushroom. Fly agarics growing in the eastern United States are yellow and not usually psychoactive. Those in the western states are red or orange; their pharmacological power correlates with cap color, the reddest mushrooms being strongest.

Amanita muscaria was the traditional intoxicant of a number of primitive tribes of Siberia — people who did not have access to other drugs but did have a shamanistic religion similar to that of many Native Americans. Publicity about the intoxicating effect of this mushroom in the 1960s led many young people in California and other western states to experiment with it as a new natural high.

People have consumed the fly agaric in many forms. The red peel of the cap, which is easily removed, can be dried and smoked. The whole mushroom can be eaten fresh, cooked, or dried; or it can be brewed into a tea and drunk. These different preparations may produce different results. Also, the mushrooms seem to vary greatly in strength and effect depending on where and when they grow and what trees they grow around.

Moderate doses cause a dreamy intoxication that some people find pleasant, but there are often uncomfortable physical symptoms. High doses can produce delirious excitement and significant toxicity. The effect comes on within thirty minutes and lasts for four to eight hours.

The responsible chemicals are ibotenic acid and muscimol, substances that resemble GABA, one of the brain's own neurotransmitters. Higher doses of them are found in a close relative of *Amanita muscaria,* a brown mushroom with white dots called the panther mushroom, or *Amanita pantherina.* It grows in woods in the Pacific Northwest and other parts of the world, and in recent years many people have also experimented with it as a way of altering consciousness.

The panther mushroom, *Amanita pantherina,* growing in the woods in western Washington State. (Jeremy Bigwood)

Again, the panther's effects are very variable, so that it may be hard to estimate a manageable dose and easy to take too much. High doses of the panther can make people very sick for up to twelve hours, and a few eaters of it have injured themselves as a result of accidents while they were delirious.

It would be foolish to experiment with either of these mushrooms without good advice from someone experienced with them about exact dose and method of preparation.

Nutmeg and Mace

Nutmeg, the ground spice that goes into cookies, eggnog, and pumpkin pie, contains a drug called myristicin that may be converted in the body to one of the amphetaminelike psychedelics. Nutmeg is the seed of a tropical tree. The outer covering of this seed is ground into a similar spice, called mace, that often flavors cakes. Both nutmeg and mace have a long history of use as psychoactive drugs, especially by people who can't obtain better ones.

To get high on nutmeg or mace you have to eat a lot of them: from a tablespoon up to a whole spice-can full. In that quantity these spices taste awful. They are also fairly toxic and regularly leave people with heavy hangovers the next day. The effects are variable, ranging from mild feelings of floating to full-blown delirium. Most people who try nutmeg out of curiosity do not come back for a second try. Frequent users are usually found only in certain prisons or other situations where more desirable drugs are unobtainable.

Some Warnings About Deliriants

1. Delirium is an abnormal condition of the brain in which mental function is temporarily deranged. A delirious person doing anything other than lying still in a safe place is a good candidate for a serious accident.
2. Never take deliriant drugs by yourself. Make sure someone not under the influence of the drug is there to watch out for you.
3. If you must experiment with jimsonweed or other nightshades, use the root rather than leaves or seeds.
4. Do not experiment with *Amanita muscaria* or *Amanita pantherina* without good advice about dose and preparation from an experienced person in the area where the mushrooms grow. Smoking the dried colored peel of these mushrooms is the mildest way of taking them.

Someone told me you could get high by eating nutmeg. So one night I choked down a whole can, which was over an ounce. After three hours, I felt light and dreamy. It was a little like a light dose of pot. However, the next morning, I had a splitting headache, my heart was racing, and my mouth was really dry. I got dizzy whenever I managed to stand up. It lasted all day. I would never eat nutmeg again. I don't even like the taste of it in food anymore.
— twenty-two-year-old man, carpenter

5. If you eat nutmeg or mace in an effort to get high, be prepared for a terrific hangover the next day.

PCP and Ketamine

The last two drugs in this chapter are strange synthetic compounds different from any other drugs. They are often called anesthetics, but unlike the general anesthetics discussed in Chapter 7, they are not depressants. In fact they stimulate the vital functions of heartbeat and respiration, even though they produce some mental effects resembling anesthesia. Other people call them psychedelics, but they are very different from those drugs, too.

PCP (Angel Dust, Peace Pill, Hog, Animal Tranquilizer, "THC," "Cannabinol")

PCP (phencyclidine) was invented in a pharmaceutical laboratory in the late 1950s and was introduced into clinical medicine in the United States in 1963 under the trade name Sernyl. It was marketed as a surgical anesthetic but did not make people unconscious in the same way as ether. Rather, it "dissociated" consciousness from the body so that patients were not bothered by surgical procedures even though they retained some kind of awareness. Enthusiasm about the medical value of PCP diminished when reports began to come in of unpleasant side effects in many patients. These reactions included strange mental states, such as feelings of being out of the body, and visual disturbances that some patients found frightening. In 1965 the drug was withdrawn from use for humans, but two years later it was reintroduced as a veterinary anesthetic under the name Sernylan. Animals could not tell their veterinarians that they disliked the side effects.

At about the same time PCP made its first appearance on the black market. It is a cheap and easy drug to make, produces a strong intoxication, and can be sold to unsuspecting buyers as other, more desirable drugs. For instance, pills of PCP have often been sold as synthetic THC, the chief component of marijuana. (In fact, synthetic THC is very rare and expensive and is almost never available on the black market.) Supermarket mushrooms, treated with PCP alone or with PCP and LSD, were sold as magic mushrooms throughout the late 1960s and early 1970s. PCP-LSD combinations have also been sold as mescaline and psilocybin.

PCP comes as both pills and a powder. The powdered form, called angel dust, can be sprinkled in joints made of marijuana or inactive herbs such as parsley, mint, and oregano; or it can be dissolved in an organic solvent and sprayed on these materials. When the solvent evaporates, it leaves an even residue of the drug. Such joints are called dusters. Some people snort angel dust, and very few inject it. By any route PCP produces distinctive effects. It causes decreased sensitivity to pain and a peculiar rubbery feeling in the legs with impaired coordination. It may also cause dizziness and nausea, flushing, sweating, and abnormal movements of the eyes.

The mental effects are very variable but often include a feeling of disconnection from the body and from external reality, apathy, disorganization of thinking, a drunklike state, and distortions of time and space perception. Overdoses can cause convulsions and coma. When it is smoked, PCP's effects come on within a few minutes, peak within five to thirty minutes, and last for four to six hours. Oral doses may last longer, and some people say they do not feel normal for up to twenty-four hours after a single oral dose.

Throughout the 1960s and early 1970s most people who took PCP took it unwittingly, thinking they were taking something else — mescaline, psilocybin, or some sort of supermarijuana. It came in all kinds of disguises. Few people took it for its own merits, and it had a not very good reputation, often being put down as "animal tranquilizer."

In more recent years, however, PCP has become even more prevalent, and some people seek it out as their drug of choice. The PCP lovers who have received most publicity are teen-agers from urban ghettos whose lives are filled with anger, frustration, and violence. Maybe they like the feeling of being cut off from the grim reality of their environment or from their own emotions. Because of heavy use of PCP by such persons, the drug has now gained a reputation for causing crime, violence, and insanity among young people. No doubt some PCP-related murders have occurred, but newspapers, predictably, have blown the drug's association with violence out of all proportion, leading to legislative hearings and stiffer laws on PCP, as well as great hysteria about a new drug menace.

There does not seem to be anything about the pharmacology of PCP that automatically makes users become violent or commit crimes. Clearly, high doses can make people agitated and confused, but tendencies to criminal violence are inherent in certain people, not in certain drugs. PCP users who are not

I've had very positive experiences with PCP, which is unusual, since everyone says it's a terrible drug . . . For years I have suffered lower back pains. Whenever I smoked PCP I felt no pain, and could even jog comfortably. Even after the drug wore off, I experienced no pain from physical activities . . . My thinking was often imaginative and lucid. I laughed a lot . . . I was taking it all the time, and people around me told me I was acting too crazily. So I stopped. Sometime, I'd like to experiment with it again to explore those physical and mental powers it seems to release in me.
— thirty-six-year-old man, screenwriter

angry and violent to begin with do not become raving lunatics after smoking angel dust. The recent rash of scare stories about PCP seems to reflect society's need to have "devil drugs" more than it does the nature of PCP.

The main arguments against PCP are that its effects seem neither very interesting nor very productive for most people. Some users take it in ways they find valuable — for example, as a social or party drug much like alcohol and downers — but many young persons take it just to get "messed up" or feel disconnected from reality. Also, the adulteration of other drugs with PCP is a deplorable practice, especially when these are sold or given to unsuspecting people.

Adverse reactions to PCP can include inability to talk or communicate, a blank stare and robotlike attitude, rigid muscles, confusion, agitation, and paranoid thinking. Heavy users sometimes develop problems with speech and memory that may last for some time after they stop taking the drug.

Ketamine (Ketalar, Ketaject, Super-K)

Ketamine is a close relative of PCP, producing very similar effects. It is a legal prescription drug intended for use as an anesthetic. Ketamine comes in small bottles as a solution to be injected into patients, either intravenously or intramuscularly.

Like PCP, ketamine produces an unusual kind of anesthesia, called a dissociative state, in which the patient's awareness becomes detached from the body and from external reality. Like PCP, ketamine has produced a number of bad reactions, since many patients become frightened when they find themselves in this unusual condition. So far, however, there has been no move to take ketamine off the market.

In recent years, a number of people have experimented with ketamine as a recreational drug, but they have been very different from PCP users, with the result that ketamine has a very different reputation and following from its notorious relative.

In the first place, all ketamine is legally manufactured. Since it is not a controlled substance, it is not closely watched, and supplies of it are easily diverted from hospitals and pharmacies into the hands of recreational users. Many of its fans are doctors who have introduced their friends, including nurses and other professionals, to the drug. Ketamine users tend to be more intelligent, more educated, older, wealthier, and much more experienced with drugs than PCP users. They are able to take exact doses of pure material.

Because ketamine comes in an injectable form and because many of its users are medical personnel, it tends to be taken by injection, usually intramuscularly. Given in this way it produces an altered state of consciousness that begins in a few minutes and lasts about half an hour. The feeling is one of dreamy, floating disconnection from external reality. Some ketamine enthusiasts like to take it while lying in sensory isolation tanks in attempts to have out-of-the-body experiences.

The fact that ketamine remains an uncontrolled substance while PCP has become the chief devil drug of the 1980s is a good illustration of how images of drugs are shaped by their users. Just as marijuana has never shaken off its association with deviants, minorities, and rebels, so PCP is now linked with an angry, violent, young segment of the population that is prone to commit crimes. PCP does not cause crime, violence, or insanity any more than marijuana causes revolutions. The pharmacology of ketamine is practically the same as that of PCP, yet ketamine users lie peacefully in dissociative states, causing no one any harm, and they tend to be mature, successful professionals.

Unfortunately, many ketamine users do not realize that they can take the drug by safer routes than injection. Ketamine liquid can be evaporated to solid crystals that can be powdered and smoked, snorted, or swallowed, just like PCP. By the oral route, ketamine lasts longer, and the peak effect is less dramatic. By any route, high doses of ketamine can be as unpleasant as high doses of PCP.

Some Suggestions About PCP and Ketamine

1. Try to avoid taking PCP unintentionally. All street psychedelics in pill or powder form are suspect, as are funny-tasting joints that give strange rushes.
2. If you take PCP deliberately, avoid high doses.
3. As with other drugs, the oral route is safer. Smoking PCP gives a rapid, dramatic effect. Some users prefer to smoke because they know right away how high they are. If you take PCP by mouth, it is even more important to know the dose so that you don't get more intoxicated than you intend.
4. Do not take PCP with depressants or stimulants. The combined effects can be unpleasant and difficult to control.
5. Because PCP affects coordination, thought, and judgment, do not do things under its influence that require those functions to be normal.
6. Because PCP can produce agitation, confusion, and difficulties in communication, it is not wise to take it in settings or with people that might add to those problems.

7. If you take PCP regularly and find you have trouble thinking clearly or remembering, cut down or stop taking it altogether.
8. If you meet people who want you to try ketamine, remember that it is essentially the same as PCP.
9. Remember also that ketamine can be taken by mouth and does not have to be injected.

Suggested Reading

Accurate information on solvent sniffing will be found in *Licit and Illicit Drugs* by Edward M. Brecher and the editors of *Consumer Reports* (Boston: Little, Brown, 1972).

There are a number of good books on plants of the nightshade family and the strange effects they produce. Charles B. Heiser's *Nightshades: The Paradoxical Plants* (San Francisco: W. H. Freeman, 1969) discusses the edible nightshades and tobacco as well as the deliriant members of the family. Harold A. Hansen's *The Witch's Garden* (Santa Cruz, California: Unity Press, 1978) concentrates on belladonna, henbane, mandrake, and datura.

Jonathan Ott includes *Amanita muscaria* and *Amanita pantherina* in his *Hallucinogenic Plants of North America* (Berkeley, California: Wingbow Press, 1976; revised edition, 1979). Descriptions of uses of *Amanita muscaria* will be found in *Narcotic Plants of the Old World, Used in Rituals and Everyday Life: An Anthology of Texts from Ancient Times to the Present*, edited by Hedwig Schleiffer (Monticello, New York: Lubrecht & Cramer, 1979). In *Soma: Divine Mushroom of Immortality* (New York: Harcourt Brace Jovanovich, 1972), R. Gordon Wasson presents his theory that *Amanita muscaria* was used as a sacramental intoxicant in ancient India.

Graphic descriptions of the effects of ketamine occur throughout John C. Lilly's autobiographical work *The Scientist: A Novel Autobiography* (Philadelphia: Lippincott, 1978).

11

Medical Drugs and Herbal Remedies

A GREAT MANY psychoactive drugs are sold legally: as prescription medicines used by doctors, as over-the-counter remedies stocked in drugstores, and as herbal products available in many health food stores. Patients and consumers are often unaware of the effects of these substances. We review the more common ones in this chapter.

I firmly believe that if the whole materia medica as now used could be sunk to the bottom of the sea, it would be all the better for mankind and all the worse for the fishes.
— Oliver Wendell Holmes (1809–1894), American physician and author

Psychiatric Drugs

Psychiatrists now rely heavily on drugs to treat the symptoms of mental illness. Although these chemicals do affect mood, perception, and thought, they rarely cause euphoria or trigger high states; as a result, people generally do not take them unless they are psychiatric patients. Psychiatric medications fall into three main categories: major tranquilizers, antidepressants, and lithium.

Major Tranquilizers (Thorazine and Relatives)
Major tranquilizers revolutionized psychiatry when they were first introduced in the early 1950s. They provided a new and easy way to manage schizophrenia and other severe mental diseases, making patients calm and emotionally quiet. In some cases the major tranquilizers have enabled psychotic persons to

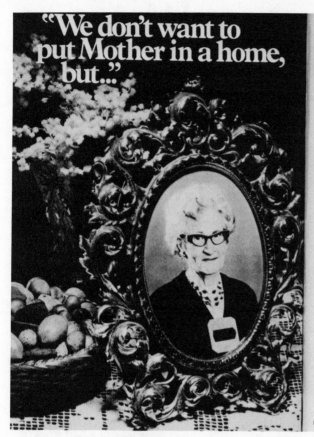

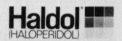

Example of an advertisement for a major tranquilizer. (Used with permission of and copyright by McNEILAB INC.)

lead reasonably normal lives and function outside hospitals. More often, they make them more manageable and docile rather than less crazy.

The most widely used drug in this group is chlorpromazine (Thorazine). Other common ones are haloperidol (Haldol), fluphenazine (Prolixin), perphenazine (Trilafon), prochlorperazine (Compazine), thioridazine (Mellaril), and trifluoperazine (Stelazine).

In addition to their use in treating mental illness, the major tranquilizers can be used to end bad reactions to psychedelic drugs and other states of confusion. Some of them are also used to treat purely physical problems, such as itching, dizziness, nausea, vomiting, and hiccups.

In normal people, small doses of these compounds cause drowsiness, lethargy, and boredom — hardly the kinds of effects that encourage recreational use. In addition, the major tranquilizers regularly produce uncomfortable physical effects, such as dryness of the mouth. In high doses and long-term use they can also cause more serious toxicity, such as liver and eye damage and permanent disorders of muscle movement and coordination.

Because the physical and mental effects of major tranquilizers are at best uninteresting and at worst very unpleasant, nonmedical use of them is extremely rare.

Antidepressants (Elavil and Relatives)

The word *antidepressant* sounds attractive. It suggests a drug that lifts mood and makes you feel good, something like a stimulant. The antidepressant drugs used in psychiatry today, however, do not give the good feelings of stimulants. Instead, they often cause sedation and a variety of uncomfortable physical effects.

These drugs date from 1958, when the parent compound, imipramine (Tofranil), was invented. It is still in wide use today, along with a close relative, amitriptyline (Elavil), and a number of other similar drugs. Some depressed patients respond very well to these medications but not until after at least two weeks of regular use. On the other hand, the toxic effects begin right away: sedation, dry mouth, blurred vision, constipation, difficulty in urinating. Normal people are likely to notice only these "side effects" without any positive mood changes.

Like the major tranquilizers, the antidepressants do not lend themselves to recreational use because no one likes their effects. Often, even depressed patients who are helped by them like to cut dosage to a minimum and do without them altogether when they can. Do not be misled by their name: antidepressants will not make you high.

Lithium (Lithane, Lithonate)

Lithium salts are a relatively new treatment for manic-depressive psychosis, a serious mental illness in which people swing back and forth between extremes of mood, from intense elation (mania) to intense depression. Lithium damps out these mood swings and is especially good at preventing manic episodes, although it is also used to treat depression. It has many side effects and can produce serious toxicity in the nervous system, heart, and kidneys. It has no effects on the mind that recommend it for nonmedical use.

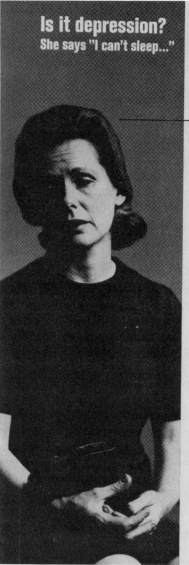

Prescription Drugs Not Commonly Thought to Be Psychoactive

Many medical drugs have mental effects that are ignored by doctors who prescribe them. Often, these effects are listed as "side effects" in the fine-print information that manufacturers include with drugs. Sometimes patients find the side effects more prominent than the main effects.

Antihistamines

Some allergic reactions are mediated by an endogenous substance called histamine that strongly affects nerves, blood vessels, and other tissues. In an effort to suppress allergic symptoms, pharmacologists have invented a number of synthetic drugs to block the actions of histamine. Many antihistamines are now available; in large-dosage forms they are dispensed by prescription, but lower-dosage forms are sold over the counter. Some of the ones in widespread use are: diphenhydramine (Benadryl), chlorpheniramine (Teldrin, Chlor-Trimeton), brompheniramine (Dimetane), dexchlorpheniramine (Polaramine), tripelennamine (PBZ, Pyribenzamine), tripolidine (Actidil), promethazine (Phenergan), pyrilamine, and doxylamine.

Although antihistamines are strong drugs that affect many systems of the body, they are often not very efficient at doing what they are supposed to do: counteract histamine and suppress allergies. The central nervous system is especially sensitive to antihistamines. Often these drugs cause profound alterations of mood, not for the better. They make people depressed, grouchy, lethargic, drowsy, and unable to think clearly. Some of them are related chemically to major tranquilizers like Thorazine, which produce similar effects on mood. The sedation caused by antihistamines may interfere with driving and other activities requiring concentration, clear thinking, and good reflexes. These effects may be intensified by the simultaneous use of alcohol and other depressants.

Despite their tendency to put people in bad moods, antihistamines are among the most widely consumed of all medical drugs, and neither doctors nor patients think of them as psychoactive. Furthermore, antihistamines are common ingredients of many over-the-counter preparations, such as cold remedies and sleeping aids; they sometimes even arrive in the mail in free samples of these products. Anyone suffering from chronic depression and lethargy should make sure they are not consuming these chemicals in one form or another. Allergy sufferers should also know that allergic symptoms frequently respond to nondrug treatments, such as changes in diet and mental state, making it possible to avoid antihistamines entirely.

A few drugs in this class are used specifically to prevent motion sickness. Dimenhydrinate (Dramamine) is the best known. Like its relatives, it often makes people drowsy and puts them in unwelcome states of mind.

Oddly enough, one antihistamine is used by some people, mostly junkies, to get high. It is tripelennamine, sold under the brand names PBZ and Pyribenzamine. Because a common form

Throughout junior high school and high school I suffered from bad hay fever. My family doctor prescribed antihistamines for me. They definitely worked, but they made me feel so bad. Finally, I came to prefer the hay fever. I was happier sneezing than being so depressed and logy. Once, while in college, I took a twenty-five-milligram tablet of Thorazine and I was amazed at how similar the effect was to the antihistamines. I hate that feeling. I managed to get rid of most of my allergies by changing my diet and lifestyle. I haven't taken an antihistamine in years.
— thirty-eight-year-old man, musician

of it is a blue tablet, it is known as "blues" on the street. The combination of morphine and blues is called "blue velvet"; some junkies like to inject it intravenously. A more popular combination is the synthetic opiate pentazocine (Talwin) and PBZ, which is known as "T's and B's" or "T's and blues" and is also taken intravenously. Except for this strange practice, recreational use of antihistamines is rare to nonexistent.

The use of antihistamines in high doses or over long periods seems unwise. These drugs have known toxicity on the physical body, and no one should spend more time than necessary in the mental states they produce.

Steroids (Cortisone and Relatives)

Besides producing adrenaline, the adrenal glands secrete other hormones that control metabolism and body chemistry. This group of hormones comes from the gland's outer layer, or cortex, and so the principal one is called cortisone. Cortisone and its relatives all have a distinctive molecular structure known as the steroid nucleus, which also occurs in male and female sex hormones. Pharmacologists have learned to make many semisynthetic drugs with this same structure, starting with raw materials found in certain plants. As a group, these drugs are all called steroids, both the endogenous ones and the manmade ones.

One of the dramatic effects of cortisone is to reduce inflammation and certain allergic reactions, such as skin rashes. Pharmacologists have maximized this action in some of the new steroids they have created in laboratories. When these drugs are applied topically — that is, when they are put on the skin — they are reasonably safe and sometimes miraculously effective. Doctors also frequently prescribe steroids for systemic use — that is, to be taken internally. There are clear indications for such use, but because steroids seem almost to have magic powers, doctors tend to overprescribe them, sometimes dispensing them for mild cases of poison ivy and other conditions not severe enough to warrant their use.

The trouble is that the desirable anti-inflammatory properties of steroids are just one of many actions of these powerful hormones. Even in moderate doses, systemic steroids can drastically upset the chemical balance of the body and cause serious toxicity, including death. They can also shut off the body's production of its own steroids with such consequences as increased susceptibility to stress and infection.

The adverse physical side effects of steroids are well known to doctors, but less attention is paid to their psychoactivity.

These drugs can produce extreme euphoria, resembling the manic phase of manic-depressive psychosis. In such cases, judgment can be severely impaired and behavior become erratic and illogical. With continued use this initial euphoria may turn into intense depression. Steroids can make some people psychotic or suicidal. Not everyone taking steroids systemically experiences these dramatic reactions, but many probably experience more subtle changes in mood; nervousness, insomnia, depression, and other mental changes are common with long-term use. People with a history of psychiatric problems should be cautious about taking steroids. Everyone should be aware that these compounds are among the strongest drugs known and so should be saved for the treatment of really serious illness.

The sex-hormone group of steroids, including estrogen and testosterone, can produce mental effects as well, although their physical toxicity is usually more serious. Female hormones are ingredients of birth-control pills, and have been prescribed in ways that now seem unwise, such as to treat normal conditions, like menopause, that should not be regarded as diseases in the first place. Some male athletes take male hormones to increase muscle bulk, a practice horrifying to anyone aware of the delicate hormonal balance of the human body.

Cough Suppressants

The oldest and most effective drugs for coughs are the opiates. They directly depress the center in the brain that controls the cough reflex. It is not always a good idea to stop people from coughing; sometimes they need to expel material from the respiratory tract. If an unproductive cough continues, however, it should be stopped.

The most common opiate prescribed for coughs is codeine, a relatively less powerful one that is reasonably active by mouth. Because of the danger of dependence, doctors do not like to prescribe opiates casually. Pharmacologists have tried to vary the molecules of opiates to come up with new compounds that will suppress coughs but not cause euphoria or dependence. Some of their inventions are available by prescription, such as hydrocodone, a semisynthetic derivative of codeine. Although these narcotic cough suppressants carry warnings about dependence, patients and doctors may not appreciate the reality of the risk until it is too late. Also, these drugs, like other narcotics, are depressants and can interfere with thinking and motor coordination. If they are the only thing that works for a bad cough, they should be taken intermittently or for only a few days in a row so as to avoid habitual use.

I've had asthma all my life and am allergic to just about everything . . . As a child I took a lot of codeine for coughs. For the past ten years I've been on Hycodan, which I understand contains a narcotic [hydrocodone]. Originally, I took one tablet four times a day; now I take two four times a day. If I try to cut down the dose I start coughing and get really congested. Also, I get upset and can't sleep.

If I think about it, I guess I know I'm addicted, but I don't like to face that. I've never had anything to do with drugs . . .
— fifty-two-year-old woman, university guidance counselor

Gastrointestinal Drugs

One of the commonest drugs used to treat intestinal cramps and diarrhea is Lomotil, a combination of a synthetic opiate called diphenoxylate and atropine, one of the constituents of nightshade plants. Both of these drugs reduce the movement of the intestines by paralyzing the nerves that control them. Diphenoxylate is a close chemical relative of meperidine (Demerol), one of the strong medical narcotics. Like its relative, diphenoxylate can cause depression of the nervous system that may be intensified by simultaneous use of other depressants. It can also cause euphoria and dependence. Many patients who take Lomotil for intestinal upset experience narcotic effects on mood but have no idea they are using an opiate.

Atropine by itself has little psychoactivity in low doses; most people find high doses unpleasant. Some combination drugs mix atropine with other nightshade derivatives, including scopolamine, the main psychoactive principle of the nightshade family. Donnatal is an example of such a mixture; it also includes some phenobarbital as a sedative. Doctors frequently maintain patients on these drugs, especially patients with ulcers, gastrointestinal spasms, and urinary disorders. Rarely do doctors or patients consider the potential of these treatments to affect mood and thought, but as noted in the section on deliriants,* nightshade drugs can influence the mind profoundly. The psychoactive effect most likely to be noticed by people who take these drugs is drowsiness, but over time, or in high dosage, they may cause more bizarre changes.

"Mild" Analgesics

Pharmacologists have been unable to come up with analgesics (pain relievers) of medium strength to fill the gap between aspirin and morphine. They have given us several derivatives of opiates that they claimed were more powerful than aspirin but safer and less addicting than morphine. If these drugs are effective at controlling pain, however, they always turn out to be attractive to opiate addicts and are likely to cause dependence.

One such drug is propoxyphene (Darvon), a prescription analgesic widely used in recent years. Sometimes it is combined with aspirin and caffeine to make it more effective. Despite enthusiastic claims of its manufacturer, most doctors and patients have found Darvon to be not much more effective than aspirin. (Some even feel that when it is combined with aspirin, it is the aspirin that does most of the work.) Besides, the abuse potential

*See pages 130–36.

of Darvon is of the same sort as that of the strong narcotic analgesics. It took some time for doctors to acknowledge the existence of Darvon abuse, but they are now very familiar with it and much more cautious about dispensing the drug.

In addition to the above categories, many other prescription drugs may have psychoactive effects, even if doctors, pharmacologists, and manufacturers don't recognize them. Sometimes these effects show up in many patients who take a drug, sometimes in only a few. If you begin a course of prescription drug treatment and experience sleepiness, depression, highs, unusual dreams, or other mental changes you cannot account for, the drug may be responsible. To prove it, you would have to stop the drug and, after an interval, start it again to see if there is a relationship between it and the symptoms.

Over-the-Counter (OTC) Preparations

Cough Syrups

OTC cough syrups are of varied composition. Some contain no obviously psychoactive drugs. Others contain known depressants, such as alcohol and chloroform; stimulants such as phenylpropanolamine; antihistamines; and derivatives of opiates considered to be nonnarcotic. Sometimes people who are desperate for drugs and who cannot get anything better consume overdoses of these preparations in efforts to get high.

The principal OTC cough suppressant is a drug called dextromethorphan, a relative of codeine that quiets the cough center but does not produce euphoria, dependence, or the other characteristic effects of narcotics. Still, it may cause drowsiness and depression of respiration.

Cold Remedies

Capsules and tablets for relieving symptoms of colds account for a large percentage of OTC drug sales. Like the cough syrups, they are a mixed bag of different formulas and strengths. Common ingredients are antihistamines, aspirin and other pain relievers, nightshade drugs to dry up excess secretion in the nose and throat, and caffeine and phenylpropanolamine to offset the sedative effects of the other ingredients. Usually these mixtures are packaged in multicolored tablets and flashy capsules to make them look exotic and powerful. Whether they affect the course of a cold or significantly reduce the symptoms is questionable. (Even when they do suppress symptoms, they may actually prolong colds by making people less aware of their illness and less likely to take good care of themselves.) What is more certain is that OTC cold remedies can affect mood, usually in undesirable ways. Alternate methods of treating colds to avoid these problems include taking hot baths, forcing fluids, eating less, increasing rest, and decreasing stress and stimulation.

Nasal Decongestants

One of the physical effects of stimulants is to constrict blood vessels in the nose and sinuses. This constriction shrinks those tissues, allowing freer passage of air. The effect is temporary and, when the stimulant wears off, is usually followed by an opposite reaction, or "rebound," in which the nasal passages become more blocked than before.

Early nasal inhalers contained strips of paper impregnated with amphetamine. Many users experienced general stimulation from them, some got high, and some became dependent. Some even broke open the containers and extracted the amphetamine in order to put it into their bodies in other ways. Eventually, manufacturers stopped using amphetamine in nasal inhalers, replacing it with other drugs supposed to be less stimulating and less addictive.

Today, the OTC inhalers and sprays sold to unblock stuffy noses are not considered psychoactive. Some of the inhalers contain no drugs but only aromatic substances such as menthol. They may be pleasant to use but are not nearly as effective as chemicals that constrict blood vessels. The sprays and those inhalers that do contain drugs certainly work in the short run, but though the manufacturers claim otherwise, they are still stimulants and frequently cause dependence.

Not everyone experiences general stimulation from these products, but those who do may come to use them habitually. Probably, a greater risk of dependence arises from the temporary nature of the relief they offer. If people continue to use them to treat the rebound that follows the initial dose, they quickly find themselves unable to breathe without them. Longer-acting preparations may be safer in this respect.

A few oral forms of decongestants are available: for example, pseudoephedrine (Sudafed), a close relative of the natural stimulant ephedrine. Since it goes into the mouth rather than the nose, it is less likely to cause rebound and dependence, but for some people and in high doses it is definitely a stimulant. Our old friend phenylpropanolamine is often identified as an

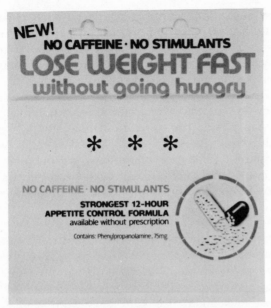

NEW!
NO CAFFEINE · NO STIMULANTS
LOSE WEIGHT FAST
without going hungry

✳   ✳   ✳

NO CAFFEINE · NO STIMULANTS
STRONGEST 12-HOUR
APPETITE CONTROL FORMULA
available without prescription
Contains: Phenylpropanolamine, 75mg

oral decongestant when it appears in OTC cold remedies and cough syrups; of course, it, too, is a stimulant.

Appetite Suppressants

We mentioned these oral forms of stimulants at the end of Chapter 6. They usually contain phenylpropanolamine, sometimes combined with caffeine, and are packaged and named to look like amphetamines.

OTC Uppers

Pure caffeine is sold in most drugstores for much more than it is worth in clever disguises meant to suggest powerful amphetamines. For example, a product called Caffedrine in large, green and white time-release capsules looks just like pharmaceutical Dexamyl. No doubt some people who buy it resell it on the black market as Dexamyl to gullible buyers. Older and more straightforward products are Vivarin and No-Doz, in the form of simple white tablets. If these products are more effective than coffee or tea, it is only because people believe in pills.

OTC Downers

A variety of products are available in drugstores to reduce anxiety during the day (Compoz, for example) or promote sleep at night (Nytol, Sominex). They are widely used as nonprescription analogs of the stronger minor tranquilizers and sleeping

This package of diet capsules emphasizes that the product contains "no stimulants." The sole active ingredient is phenylpropanolamine, a stimulant.

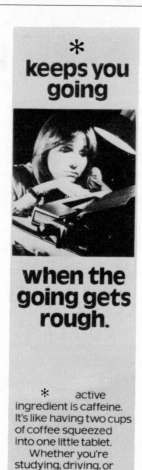

This ad for caffeine in tablet form appeared in several women's magazines.

pills. All of them contain antihistamines, usually pyrilamine or doxylamine. As we have pointed out, these chemicals are not innocuous and tend to affect mental function in unpleasant ways. They will make people drowsy but can produce depression as well and can be habit-forming.

We favor less toxic remedies for insomnia, such as increased exercise during the day, decreased use of stimulants, especially in the evening (remember to read labels of any pain pills, cold tablets, and other remedies to see if they contain caffeine or other stimulants), relaxation techniques, warm baths, and simple nutritional supplements such as calcium and magnesium tablets, which relax many people when taken at bedtime.

Analgesics

Although nonnarcotic pain relievers do not directly affect the mind, they can change moods dramatically by decreasing discomfort and so can be habit-forming. The common OTC analgesics, such as aspirin and acetaminophen (Tylenol), are effective remedies for occasional use, but when pain persists, people should seek to identify and treat the causes rather than rely on these drugs. Some analgesic compounds contain caffeine solely for its stimulant and mood-elevating effects.

OTC drugs are big business and are not regulated in the same way as prescription drugs. Manufacturers can get them on the market without doing much to prove their effectiveness, can deemphasize their adverse effects, and can make outrageous claims in their advertising. Most people assume that the products heaped on drugstore counters are mild but effective, nontoxic, and nonaddictive. Those are not safe assumptions. Anyone who uses OTC drugs should know what they contain and how they affect the body and mind.

Herbal Remedies

With increasing interest in alternatives to regular medicine, the marketing of herbal remedies and medicinal plants has boomed. Most health food stores have herb departments, and some of the products they sell are even appearing in drugstores and supermarkets. Many are just pleasant herbal teas, such as peppermint and chamomile, without significant drug effects, but a few are really psychoactive. In Chapter 6, we discussed guaraná, maté, yohimbe, and ephedra, all stimulants.

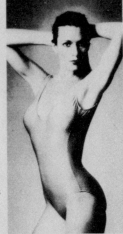
A plant with the opposite effect is valerian; its root is a strong natural sedative that does not depress vital functions or cause the kind of dependence that sleeping pills do. Preparations of valerian root, including tinctures and capsules, are obtainable at health food stores. Valerian has a strange, musty odor that some people find disagreeable, but it is easy to take as a capsule or tincture and does work. For people who need nighttime sedatives, it is probably a better choice than more dangerous, synthetic drugs.

Kava, or kava-kava, is another herbal depressant whose effect is of a more general anesthetic nature than a sedative. It is the root of a large tropical plant related to black pepper and

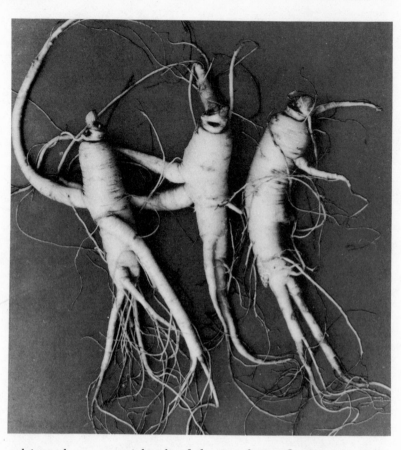

Ginseng roots.

cultivated on many islands of the South Pacific. Natives there make drinks from fresh or dried kava root and consume them as ritual and social drugs. Preparations of the fresh root are more powerful, putting users into pleasant, dreamy states while numbing their bodies. Drinks made from the dried root are more relaxing than intoxicating. Kava ceremonies take place at night and often bring large groups of people together for the main social event of island life. Only dried kava is available outside the South Pacific. Herb stores sell it as a coarse powder or larger chips of root. When chewed, dried kava makes the mouth numb and may be relaxing. Some people brew it into a tea, which they like as a mild downer.

One of the most famous of the plant drugs is ginseng, obtained from the roots of several species of woodland plants, one from China and Korea and another from the northeastern United States. People in the Orient have used ginseng for centuries, paying high prices for the best quality roots and valuing them as general tonics. They believe ginseng increases vitality, resistance to disease, and longevity. It is especially used by men, and those who use it often say it increases sexual power, particularly as they grow older.

Ginseng has only recently become popular in the West, and Western scientists still do not understand it very well. They are convinced that ginseng has effects, but they don't yet know what all of them are. One source of confusion is that commercial products vary tremendously in potency, some having no activity at all. For some people ginseng is a strong stimulant. It may raise blood pressure and should be used with caution by people with high blood pressure. Other users claim it tones their muscles and skin and increases physical endurance. "Siberian ginseng" is not true ginseng but comes from a related plant; it may be less of a stimulant.

Effects of ginseng are cumulative, often not becoming apparent unless the drug is used regularly for weeks or months. The chemistry of the root is very complex. Some compounds in it may affect the production of steroid hormones, which could explain the results users report. In any case, ginseng is a drug, not just a dietary supplement or new-age hoax, even though it now appears in everything from toothpaste to soda. If you want to try ginseng, avoid these senseless preparations and be prepared to spend a lot of money for whole roots, capsules, or extracts of reliable potency.

Suggested Reading

There are a number of guides to medical drugs written for patients. Three useful ones are: *The Doctors and Patients Handbook of Medicines and Drugs* by Peter Parish (second edition, revised; New York: Knopf, 1980); *The Essential Guide to Prescription Drugs* by James W. Long (revised edition; New York: Harper & Row, 1980); and *Pills That Don't Work: A Consumer's and Doctor's Guide to Over 600 Prescription Drugs That Lack Evidence of Effectiveness* by Sidney M. Wolfe, Christopher M. Coley, and the Health Research Group founded by Ralph Nader (New York: Farrar, Straus & Giroux, 1981). All these books are written by medical doctors.

Is There No Place on Earth for Me? by Susan Sheehan (Boston: Houghton Mifflin, 1982) is a vivid case history of a young schizophrenic woman, who, during repeated hospitalizations, is "treated" with ever-increasing doses of virtually all the major tranquilizers currently in use.

Two of the best reference books on herbal medicine are *Potter's New Cyclopaedia of Medicinal Herbs and Preparations*, edited by R. W. Wren (New York: Harper & Row, 1972); and *A Modern Herbal* (in two volumes) by Mrs. M. Grieve (New York: Dover, 1971).

12

Problems with Drugs

IN THE PRECEDING CHAPTERS we have discussed the risks and problems associated with using specific drugs. Here we will comment on some more general problems drug users are apt to encounter.

Uncertainty of Dose and Quality

When drugs come from legal sources they are likely to be pure, of standard dosage, and correctly labeled. Yet even medical drugs can be outdated and mislabeled, and they sometimes contain fillers and colorings that can be harmful to some people. These problems are insignificant compared to those of black-market drugs, which are regularly cut with impurities, are of uncertain dosage, and are often completely misrepresented to the buyer.

Buying pills and powders on the street is a risky business at best. Not only do you have to deal with unsavory characters and participate in illegal transactions, you have no assurance of getting what you pay for. If you are lucky, what you buy will contain some of what it's supposed to contain and be cut with nothing more dangerous than starch or sugar. If you are less lucky, the pills and powders will be inactive, and if you aren't lucky at all, they will contain something actively harmful. Not only are you likely to get ripped off on the black market, you can also wind up in a hospital emergency room. People who inject street

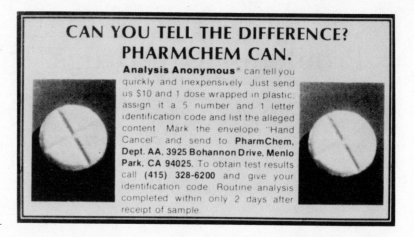

(Courtesy of PharmChem Laboratories)

drugs are in greatest danger, because putting impurities directly into the bloodstream gives the body no chance to deal with them.

Even natural drugs are suspect on the black market. Marijuana may be laced with PCP or contaminated with paraquat. "Magic mushrooms" may be very ordinary mushrooms sprayed with LSD or PCP, and even if they are the genuine article, it is impossible to know how potent they are.

Some help with these uncertainties is offered by private testing labs that will analyze samples of drugs for a reasonable fee while protecting the customer's anonymity. Drug enforcement authorities will not allow these labs to give quantitative results, however, so that although you may find out what is in your material, you still won't know how potent it is. About the only way to be sure that you are getting what you want in the way of nonmedical drugs is to grow your own drug plants or collect them in the wild. Otherwise, try to know your sources; remember that the black market encourages deception and misrepresentation, and be extremely cautious about consuming any substance obtained on the street.

Mixing Drugs

In a few instances, the results of mixing psychoactive drugs are clear. For example, we have noted the additive effects of combining alcohol and downers or tranquilizers. In many more cases the effects of drug combinations are unpredictable, depending more on the individual and on set and setting than on pharmacology. Mixing drugs can increase the problems associated with individual drugs and may create some new ones.

At the very least, drug combinations take getting used to. Many marijuana smokers use alcohol while smoking, but there is no predictable result of this combination. Some people find themselves more stoned, others less stoned, others sleepy or headachy. Until you know the effects of a given combination on *you*, you should proceed cautiously. People who get into bad relationships with drugs often use many drugs together, and some combinations may promote dependency and abuse. People who ingest alcohol and cocaine together often wind up taking more of both than they would if they used either by itself. Coffee and cigarettes together form a very stubborn habit — it is almost as if one triggers a desire for the other.

These days it is not unusual to see groups of people drinking alcohol, snorting coke, and smoking pot, as well as using tobacco, drinking coffee, and eating chocolate — all at the same time and in large doses. Such polydrug consumption is not necessarily harmful on occasion, but it tends to promote immoderation and lack of awareness about the nature of the substances being consumed.

Drug combining is a problem in medicine as well. Medical patients often receive many prescription drugs simultaneously, and doctors are often ignorant about how they interact. Interactions of medical drugs and recreational drugs are also largely unknown. If you are taking medical drugs, keep in mind that they might change your reaction to recreational drugs. If you use recreational drugs, consider that they might combine unfavorably with prescribed medication.

Medical Problems

Acute Problems

Overdosing and allergic reactions are the most important acute medical problems that can arise from taking psychoactive drugs. Mild overdoses of drugs may produce nausea and vomiting, which usually require no treatment but can be very unpleasant. Large overdoses can cause convulsions, coma, and death; they are medical emergencies requiring immediate treatment in hospitals. Anyone who suddenly loses consciousness or stops breathing after taking a drug should be seen immediately by a doctor. If you are around someone who develops an overdose (OD) reaction, put all legal considerations aside and summon medical help. Never administer more drugs — of *any* type — to a person suffering from overdose.

Intravenous users of drugs are in the greatest danger of dramatic overdose reactions, but people who smoke or snort stimulants and depressants can have them too, as can people who take very large doses by mouth. Remember that ODs can quickly result in death if hospital treatment is not obtained immediately.

Allergic reactions to drugs take many forms, ranging from itching and swelling of parts of the body to death from asphyxiation owing to the swelling of tissues in the windpipe. Serious allergic reactions are very unpredictable and may occur to contaminants of street drugs as well as to the drugs themselves. They may also develop suddenly in people with no prior history of allergy. The symptoms of serious allergic shock are itching in the throat and difficulty in breathing. Again, this is a medical emergency requiring prompt treatment. Anyone who develops such a reaction should be taken to a hospital at once.

Chronic Medical Problems

Any drug used in excess over time can produce illness. Different drugs irritate different systems of the body. In some cases the association between a drug and a disease is very clear, as it is with alcohol and cirrhosis of the liver or tobacco in the form of cigarettes and lung cancer. In other cases it is simply speculative, as with coffee and pancreatic cancer. We have reviewed these specific physical consequences in previous chapters.

People who use any drug intravenously expose themselves to other risks that are consequences of that method of administration. Putting crude and unsterilized needles into veins carries a grave danger of introducing serious infections. Hepatitis is probably the most common disease transmitted in this way; it can make people sick for months and cause permanent liver damage. Less common but more serious is bacterial endocarditis — an infection of the heart valves. In addition, needle users frequently suffer from abscesses and inflamed and damaged veins. Intramuscular and subcutaneous injections are less dangerous but not without risk. They transmit hepatitis equally well.

Smoking anything irritates the throat, bronchial tubes, and lungs. In susceptible individuals regular smoking of any drug, whether it is tobacco, marijuana, or cocaine, can result in respiratory infections, decreased breathing capacity, coughing, bronchitis, and, probably, a greater risk of emphysema and lung cancer. It is also important to keep in mind that smoking puts drugs into the bloodstream and brain very directly, even faster than intravenous injection, making the drugs more toxic and more addicting. Snorting drugs is less direct than intravenous injection, but not nearly as safe as oral use; it can lead to chronic irritation and erosion of the nasal membranes. Even taken by mouth, some drugs in excess are very irritating. Heavy drinking can cause chronic inflammation of the esophagus and stomach, and too much coffee often gives rise to chronic indigestion.

Heavy users of drugs often have erratic lifestyles that interfere with regular sleep, good nutrition, and healthful habits of hygiene and exercise. In addition, the drugs they take may suppress appetite, rob the body of vitamins, and upset normal metabolism. All of these effects can lead to such chronic problems as malnutrition, anemia, and decreased resistance to infection. For example, dietary deficiencies in the alcoholic greatly increase the liver's susceptibility to the toxicity of alcohol and contribute to the development of cirrhosis.

Drugs and Pregnancy

Women expose their unborn babies to harm by consuming drugs — any drugs — during pregnancy. Many doctors now advise that expectant mothers take no drugs whatever during the first three months of pregnancy and as few as possible thereafter. Psychoactive drugs are no exception. In the 1960s thousands of badly deformed babies were born to women who took the sedative thalidomide, prescribed as a "safe" relaxant and promoter of sleep.

Recreational drugs can also be risky to the fetus, but in most cases the exact dangers are unknown. It is known that mothers who smoke cigarettes have more miscarriages and regularly give birth to babies that weigh less than normal, are more susceptible to respiratory infections, and die more frequently in infancy. Drinking alcohol during pregnancy also increases the rate of birth defects; unfortunately, no one can say what a safe intake of alcohol is for a pregnant woman.

Most of the drugs discussed in this book enter the system of the fetus and affect it in some way. For example, pregnant heroin addicts give birth to addicted babies who must be weaned off opiates in the first few days of life. Given these facts, pregnant women should make an effort to discontinue the use of all psychoactive substances until after they deliver. Even then, they should be careful if they breast-feed, because if they take drugs, their milk may contain high enough amounts to affect a baby.

Smoking around an infant can also put drugs into its system, and babies are very sensitive to smoke of all sorts.

Psychiatric Problems

The most common acute psychiatric problem is panic. Typically, people will take a drug, feel it begin to work, and become convinced that they are dying or losing their minds. Panic reactions occur most frequently in people with little drug experience, especially in settings that encourage anxiety. A teen-ager who has never smoked marijuana and is pressured into trying it at a party with strangers is a good candidate for a panic reaction. People who are slipped drugs unawares, or who wind up taking much larger doses than they are used to, are also likely to panic. Panic can be very dramatic, making people agitated, helpless, incoherent, and sources of great anxiety to others. People in panic often use the anxiety they produce in others to fuel their own reactions.

Doctors have sometimes misdiagnosed panic reactions as episodes of psychosis and have prolonged them by confirming patients' fears of going crazy. People who are panicked need to be reassured and calmed down, preferably by someone with experience, such as a worker at a drug crisis center. They should not be given sedatives, tranquilizers, or other psychoactive drugs. A hospital emergency room may not be the best place to take people in panic, because it can produce more anxiety than reassurance. Most panic reactions will end quickly, provided they are recognized for what they are and not intensified by improper management.

Paranoia and "bad trips" are similar to panic reactions and are also mostly products of set and setting. They, too, will subside by themselves if left to run their course.

True psychotic reactions are occasionally triggered by drug experiences, but they are not nearly so common as panic reactions. Just as a first sexual experience, or going away from home to college, or losing a job can trigger psychosis, so can a stressful drug experience. A person who becomes mentally disturbed after taking a drug and who continues to be disturbed after the effects of the drug wear off should be seen by a professional.

Coming down from drugs ("crashing") presents special problems. People who rely on drugs to feel good may become depressed when the drugs wear off. Not only can this depression encourage frequent and abusive drug-taking, but it can also become a chronic psychological problem. Psychiatrists these days often see severely depressed patients who are heavy users of cocaine, and similar depression can occur with the regular use of any psychoactive drug. It is often a component of dependence on alcohol and downers, as well as dependence on stimulants.

Crusaders against drugs like to cite many other chronic psychological problems that are supposed to be drug-connected, but there is little evidence to support most of their claims. There does seem to be a pharmacological basis for the paranoia and hallucinations that occur in people who shoot amphetamines, and alcohol certainly can cause brain damage, producing distinctive losses of mental function. Heavy use of cocaine may cause personality changes in the direction of irritability, paranoia, and hostility. Major psychological problems may also go hand in hand with heavy consumption of other drugs, but whether they are direct effects of the drugs is seldom clear.

As an example, there has been much talk of "burn-outs" — young people who are supposed to be casualties of intense use of marijuana, psychedelics, and other illegal drugs. Certainly, there are people who wind up as aimless, confused misfits after using a lot of drugs, but what were these people like before, and what other factors played a role in the change? Many of them lived in communes, engaged in unusual sexual experimentation, or joined religious cults in addition to taking drugs. It is easy to blame the drugs, but evidence for their causative role is lacking.

An even better example of the false linking of a problem with a drug is the amotivational syndrome. As we have said, it makes much more sense to view heavy marijuana smoking as an expression of amotivation rather than the cause of it. Many amotivated people smoke a lot of marijuana, but so do many well-motivated people. Amotivated people would probably behave in other unproductive ways if marijuana were to disappear. The tendency to see disliked drugs as causes of disapproved behavior is understandable, but it is not valid scientifically and does not help solve the real problems associated with drugs.

Social Problems

Drug-taking can lead to a variety of problems with other people. Many drug users feel guilty about their habits and their guilt is often an obstacle to intimacy. Using illegal drugs automatically puts people into conflict with social authorities and with parents and teachers. One of the commonest sources of family tension today is the suspicion or discovery by parents that a child is using drugs. This issue is so emotional that most people are unable to deal with it openly. Often it creates a climate of distrust and misunderstanding that pervades every aspect of the family's life. Drug use may also isolate children from the mainstream of their peers, driving them into the company of other drug users and limiting their possibilities for balanced social interaction. Of course, children are not the only ones who encounter social problems as a result of drug use. Different preferences in recreational drugs are frequently a source of conflict in couples and can even result in breakups of marriages.

People who abuse drugs, whether legal or illegal, usually find themselves in social trouble on all levels. The alcoholic father who can't provide for his family and antagonizes his friends and coworkers is a classic example. The heroin addict who steals a friend's television set to buy his next fix is another. In fact, it is rare to find a drug abuser who does not provoke some degree of social conflict.

The drug laws in our society compound the social problems of people who choose to use illegal drugs. For one, illegal drugs are very expensive; buying them regularly can significantly drain a person's economic resources. Second, although casual users of illegal drugs generally obtain their supplies from friends, at some point the lines of supply connect to the criminal underworld. Heavy users are apt to be drawn into this sphere, especially if they begin to sell illicit substances to support their own drug habits.

The dangers of associating with professional drug dealers cannot be overstated. Many dealers handle large sums of cash, carry guns, and live in a paranoid world of rip-offs, busts, and informers. Those who grow or smuggle drugs on a large scale are also likely to be caught up in cops-and-robbers confrontations. The ugliness of drug dealing is a direct consequence of laws that criminalize the possession and sale of disapproved substances. Narcotics agents who enforce these laws sometimes behave as disreputably as the people they try to catch, violating civil liberties and recklessly employing violence to chase down "drug traffickers."

Unfortunately, major traffickers are seldom touched by the law, because they are usually rich enough, smart enough, and powerful enough to stay in business. Instead, drug-law enforcement falls disproportionately on small-scale dealers and users. In recent years, so much enforcement has been directed at these

I guess my drug of choice is wine. Two glasses of good wine put me in just the right state after a trying day. John drinks wine, too, but for getting high he prefers marijuana.

In the past few years, our different preferences in drugs have become a problem for us. My not liking marijuana separates me from John's closest friends and weakens our relationship. I don't think married people have to do everything together, but this is something important, and my inability to share John's highs bothers me. Also, I find I resent his smoking friends, since I'm the outsider, the "straight wife," when they are around. Yet I know that if I object, I will just drive him out of the house to get high with them elsewhere.

—thirty-five-year-old housewife

people that our court and prison systems are now severely over-loaded. It is also hard to avoid the suspicion that many police officers would rather go after users and dealers of illegal drugs than after more dangerous criminals.

Quite another sort of problem arises from associating with people who are intoxicated on drugs, whether legal or illegal. Intoxication increases the likelihood of accidents and trouble of all kinds. If you keep company and go out in public with drugged friends, you may suffer for their blunders.

Drunk drivers are as dangerous to their passengers and other people on the road as they are to themselves. You have a choice whether to accept rides with them, as you do with drivers who are stoned on pot, tripping on psychedelics, or under the influence of any other drugs that might compromise driving skills. It can be very difficult to refuse rides with friends because you feel they are too intoxicated, but learning to exercise that choice may save you from injury or death. In Sweden, where alcoholism is common and driving-while-intoxicated laws are strictly enforced, social custom dictates that one member of a group attending a party abstain from drinking in order to be the driver for the evening. Since our society does not have a similar custom, individuals who associate with drug users must learn to judge when they should go their separate ways.

Money is the main reason why my friends and I deal drugs. Also, there's a lot of status in it. I mean, if you've got money and drugs you've automatically got power and prestige. People say you're crazy to take the risk, but at the same time they're envious of you, and that's the truth.
— seventeen-year-old boy

Developmental Problems

The use of drugs by younger and younger children is very alarming to grownups. In the 1960s, college students were the main consumers of marijuana; today, pot is commonplace in high schools and, in some parts of the country, even in grade schools. Significant numbers of adolescents have now tried cocaine, alcohol, tobacco, tranquilizers, solvents, psychedelics, and probably more. Drugs have become prevalent in rural as well as urban schools and seem to cut across all class and ethnic boundaries.

Parents, teachers, doctors, and lawmakers generally assume that drug use by young children is especially dangerous. They fear it will cause permanent physical and psychological damage as well as create whole generations of addicts, criminals, and zombies. It may well be that children are more susceptible to the adverse effects of psychoactive drugs, but there is little hard evidence on this point. Among Native American groups who use drugs ritually, children are often introduced to natural psychedelics at very young ages without suffering any apparent harm. However, the social context of psychedelic use among these peoples is different from anything that exists in mainstream society.

Child psychologists say that adolescence is, at best, a difficult time during which children must grapple with a host of problems and pressures, some caused by internal hormonal changes, others by the changing expectations of society as they approach maturity. One concern of psychologists is that the addition of drugs into this already turbulent process will make it significantly harder. Another concern is that some children will use drugs to avoid facing the conflicts that must be resolved if they are to develop into healthy adults. At the moment there are no studies of adults who began using marijuana and other drugs while they were children. Possibly when such studies are done, the results will allay some of the worst fears. However, until then, it is no doubt safer to assume that children *are* at greater risk, and that below a certain age, drug-taking may impair normal mental and emotional development. At the very least, using psychoactive drugs in childhood to avoid boredom, conflict, and other bad feelings is likely to establish unhealthy patterns of drug-taking that will persist and cause problems in later life.

Legal Problems

I have been a criminal ever since the day I smoked my first joint.
— forty-year-old man, landscape architect

To think that a man should be allowed a gun and not a drug!
— Alexander Trocchi, from his novel Cain's Book *(1960)*

Getting arrested for possession of drugs can be devastating. At best, it can absorb a great deal of time and money; at worst, it can subject you to the horrors of prison and leave a permanent blot on your record. Current drug laws are products of society's fears and prejudices and would certainly strike an unbiased observer as irrational, if not insane. In some states, people convicted for small-scale dealing of drugs such as cocaine and LSD are treated more harshly by the law than rapists, armed robbers, and even murderers. We think that the drug laws have done much more harm than good, but the fact is they exist and are enforced. Because of diminishing public funds, the rise of violent crime, and a growing acceptance of many recreational drugs, especially marijuana, the casual user runs much less risk of arrest today than ever before. Still, law enforcement is capricious, and if you choose to use illegal drugs you always run some risk of being caught.

Although laws on possession of small amounts of marijuana have eased in many states, laws on possession with intent to sell and on trafficking in marijuana and other drugs have become more severe. Many people who share small amounts of drugs with friends are considered dealers by the law and would be subject to heavy penalties if convicted.

If you run afoul of the drug laws, waste no time in getting the advice and help of a lawyer who specializes in this area. If you have no idea where to turn for information and have little or no money, contact a local office of the Legal Aid Society, which is listed in the telephone directories of most cities. Legal Aid can advise you and help you find a lawyer.

Dependency and Addiction

A chief characteristic of a bad relationship with a drug is difficulty in leaving it alone. Dependence on drugs is common and provokes so much censure and fear that it makes it hard to see that dependence is a basic human problem not limited to drugs. People can become dependent on many substances and practices; sources of pleasure are obviously the most frequent: food, sex, drugs. People can also become dependent on certain experiences, such as falling in love or surfing, seeking them out compulsively to the exclusion of other activities. It is also easy for people to become dependent on other people. Such personal relationships share many features of drug dependence, including tolerance (diminished pleasure with frequent exposure) and withdrawal (difficulty separating). People become dependent on jogging, gambling, watching television, shopping, working, talking on the telephone, and traveling. These observations suggest that dependence has more to do with human beings than with drugs. When people talk about the "addictive potential" of a substance, what they are really talking about is the tendency of human beings to get addicted to it.

The terms *addiction* and *dependence* are used loosely today. Properly speaking, drug addiction is a special kind of dependence marked by physical changes: tolerance that requires increasing doses of the drug to achieve the same effect and a withdrawal syndrome if the drug is discontinued. People who become dependent on marijuana do not show tolerance and withdrawal as heroin addicts do. This fact has led many experts to talk about "psychological dependence." However, psychological dependence is a fuzzy concept. How does it differ from doing something repeatedly because you like it? Is there anything wrong with doing something you like repeatedly if it does not hurt you?

The real problem with dependence is that it limits personal freedom. Of course, everyone is dependent on food, water, and other people; no one can ever be completely independent. Dependencies become problems when they take up vast amounts of time, money, and energy; create guilt and anxiety; and control one's life. It is easy for people to ignore the extent to which dependencies control their lives; sometimes other people can see the problem more clearly.

Dependence on anything is not easy to break. More often than not, people simply switch dependencies, substituting one for another without achieving greater freedom. Still, it is no doubt better to be dependent on exercising, say, than on watching TV. Perhaps the tendency to become dependent is incurable, but to a certain extent people can choose what they are dependent on. Tobacco addicts who give up smoking by becoming compulsive joggers may not be any freer, but they may live longer and feel better.

Dependence on drugs may be better than dependence on some things and worse than dependence on others, but such value judgments are difficult to make without reference to particular individuals and situations. Is it better to be dependent on skydiving or snorting coke? On masturbating or eating chocolate? On fighting or shooting heroin?

Good relationships with drugs do not involve dependence. Once you become dependent on a drug it may be difficult or impossible to get back into a good relationship with it. Most experts on alcoholism say that alcoholics cannot learn to be social drinkers; their only choice is between continued alcoholism and abstinence. Most people who smoke cigarettes nonaddictively never were addicted smokers; they formed good relationships with cigarettes and maintained them. The surest way to avoid dependence on drugs is never to use them. If you do use drugs and want to avoid becoming dependent, you will have to take steps to create good relationships with them from the start.

Suggested Reading

The autobiographical books listed in the Suggested Reading sections of preceding chapters give firsthand descriptions of problems with various drugs.

Two books written for a high-school audience are *Our Chemical Culture: Drug Use and Misuse* and *Drugs: A Multimedia Sourcebook for Young Adults*, which are discussed in the Suggested Reading section for Chapter 4. For a fictional account of drug dependence among high-school students, see *Go Ask Alice* (New York: Avon Books, 1972), which was made into a television movie.

In our society, women are especially vulnerable to drug dependence. An enlightening discussion of the reasons for their vulnerability can be found in *The Female Fix* by Muriel Nellis (Boston: Houghton Mifflin, 1980).

Some insight into the dangers of drug dealing and smuggling is provided by two entertaining books of true-life adventure: Robert Sabbag's *Snowblind: A Brief Career in the Cocaine Trade* (New York: Bobbs-Merrill, 1976) and Jerry Kamstra's *Weed* (New York: Harper & Row, 1974), which concerns marijuana. The film *Midnight Express* presents a horrifying story of the consequences of getting busted for drug smuggling abroad.

For an analysis of how our drug laws create more problems than they solve, see *The Honest Politician's Guide to Crime Control* by Norval Morris and Gordon Hawkins (Chicago: University of Chicago Press, 1969). A readable history of how those laws came into being is given in *The American Disease: Origins of Narcotic Control* by David F. Musto (New Haven, Connecticut: Yale University Press, 1973).

13

Alternatives to Taking Drugs

A S WE MENTIONED at the beginning of this book, the main reason people take psychoactive drugs is to satisfy a basic human need to vary normal experience. Even very young children seem to need highs and experiment with techniques of achieving them. Why should high states be so attractive and what do drugs have to do with them?

There is growing evidence that high states are crucial to well-being. People who learn to change their conscious experience in safe and positive ways seem to be the better for it. They are healthier physically and mentally, more creative and productive, contribute more to society, and are more fun to be around. We believe that it is good to be high and important to learn good techniques to feel that way.

Being high does not mean being drugged. Clearly, drugs can sometimes make people feel high. But why is it that many persons achieve high states without ever taking drugs, and why do the people who take the most drugs lose the very effects they seek? The answer is that *drugs do not contain highs*. Highs exist within the human nervous system; all drugs do is trigger highs or provide an excuse to notice them.

That people cannot feel high whenever they want is one of the curious frustrations of the human condition. It seems necessary to work for highs, or find tools outside ourselves to evoke them. Drugs do this by making people feel temporarily different. They directly affect the nervous system and physical body in obvious ways. For example, stimulants make people feel wakeful and energized, and psychedelics alter body sensations and perceptions. Different drugs have different pharmacological effects, and so make people feel different in different ways.

No drug makes a person high automatically. One must learn to interpret the physical effects of drugs as the occasions for highs. It is expectations of individuals and society (set and setting) that encourage people to associate inner experiences with the physical feelings drugs produce. If this association fails to develop or breaks down, people can take the largest imaginable doses of drugs and not get high — just feel drugged. This is precisely the problem of those who get into bad relationships with drugs by taking them too frequently: as the novelty of the drug's effect diminishes with repetition, it no longer produces the needed signal for a high. First experiences are so powerful because the novelty of the change is greatest.

It is very easy to confuse the signal with the desired experience, the drug with the high. Many drug users are convinced that the experiences they need and like come from outside themselves in the form of drinks, joints, pills, and powders. It is this confusion that leads people to abuse drugs; they take more drugs more frequently in pursuit of ever-vanishing highs.

The fact that highs exist within is a cause for optimism. It means that the potential for high states is always there and many techniques must exist for eliciting them. There really *are* alternatives to drugs, because drug highs differ from other highs only in superficial ways. One day scientists will understand what goes on in the brain when people feel high. It may be that high states are actually mediated by the brain's own neurochemicals, which can be stimulated equally by many different influences, including one's own thoughts. Everyone has had the experience of being rocketed out of a gloomy state by a word of praise, a demonstration of affection, or the arrival of a cheering letter in the mail. That change in mood might be exactly the same on the cellular level as the rapid euphoria that follows a snort of cocaine. In fact, it might not be accurate to talk about "natural" highs, as opposed to "drug" highs, since both may depend on the body's endogenous drugs.

Is it any better to get high without drugs than with them? The main advantage of drugs over other techniques is that they can work powerfully and immediately. *Their main disadvantage*

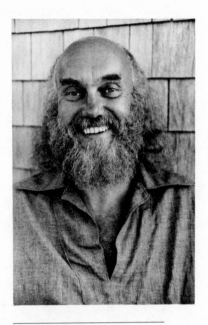

Ram Dass, formerly Richard Alpert, who, along with Timothy Leary, experimented extensively with LSD, psilocybin, and other psychedelics in the 1960s. Although an enthusiastic promoter of psychedelics when he was on the faculty at Harvard, Ram Dass later came to feel that his drug experiences were an obstacle to self-realization and that yoga and meditation were more valuable techniques. (Peter Simon)

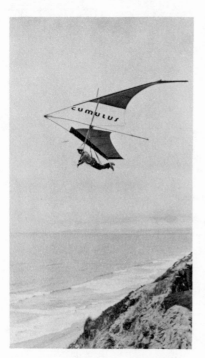

Hang-gliding over Fort Funston Bluffs, San Francisco. (Lee Foster, Free Lance Photographers Guild)

is that they reinforce the notion that the state we desire comes from something outside us. Not only can this idea lead to trouble with drugs, but it can also make people feel inadequate and incomplete. Even those in the best relationships with drugs often feel some degree of guilt about relying on them. Perhaps this feeling is so common because most people doubt their own worth and fear their abilities are not sufficient to meet the demands of life. Needing drugs to feel high confirms such fears. In any case, feeling guilty can't be good.

Of course, nondrug highs can present the same problems. People who are dependent on falling in love for their highs are equally at the mercy of outside forces. Many individuals get a rush from making money, and their lives are consumed in its pursuit. We have seen fanatical joggers who experience severe mental and physical discomfort if circumstances prevent them from running for even a day — a kind of withdrawal syndrome painful to them and those around them. If the only effective way you have of getting high is downhill skiing or hang-gliding, you are going to have to spend as much time and money getting high as any serious drug user, and will expose yourself to equal or greater physical risk. There are men who get their greatest highs from killing; some of them find acceptable roles in society as professional soldiers, others become criminals and terrorists.

The goal should be to learn how to get high in ways that do not hurt yourself or others, and that do not necessarily require huge expenditures of time or money for special materials and equipment. Furthermore, you should be able to get high in enough different ways so that you can have the experience wherever you are, even if your external resources are minimal. You should also be willing to experiment with new methods of getting high as you mature and change.

Meditation, chanting, prayer, communing with nature, playing music, and artistic expression of all sorts are especially attractive ways of changing consciousness because they require little outside oneself. This is not to say that you shouldn't play polo if playing polo gets you high, but it would be useful to have some simpler, cheaper method in your repertory as well.

Ways of getting high without drugs often do not work as fast or as powerfully as popping a pill; to master them you may have to invest some time and effort. Many people may have little motivation to acquire these skills, especially since society does not stress the value of being high or teach us practical ways to get there. People who use drugs regularly may have to work especially hard to get high in other ways, because they often grow accustomed to the physical sensations of their drugs and consider them necessary components of the experience. People who use dilute forms of drugs infrequently and by mouth will find it easier to appreciate other kinds of highs than people who put more concentrated drugs into their bodies more directly and more often, because they will not have learned to identify highs with intense pharmacological effects.

If getting high by simple methods takes more initial work, it may be worth it in the long run, because the simple methods do not fail with repeated use. In fact, methods requiring no external aids become more effective with practice. People who exercise, meditate, or do yoga to get high usually report that their experiences get better and better over time, which is a great contrast to the reports of heavy users of drugs.

There are so many ways to get high that it is not worth trying to list them. Methods that work for some people may leave others cold. We know people who have learned to get high through Sufi dancing — a grown-up version of the spinning children love — and others who find this produces nothing more than motion sickness. Contact sports give some people terrific highs, but offend the sensibilities of others. Some methods may have more followers or seem more glamorous, but the only issue of any importance is whether they work for you.

As we have noted, people also take drugs for other reasons than getting high, and alternatives exist for these as well. For instance, it isn't necessary to take drugs to treat disease; many drugless systems of therapy exist, such as acupuncture, massage, and regulation of diet. Moods can be altered and performance improved by changing patterns of eating, sleeping, and exercise. Creativity can be stimulated by traveling, reading books, talking to people, and having new experiences. You can explore your mind with the aid of psychotherapy, hypnosis, or writing or singing about your inner experiences. Since the use of drugs has become so habitual in connection with certain activities (a glass of wine with dinner, a joint before a movie), it may be hard for some people to imagine life without them. The fact is, however, that if people are determined enough, they can eliminate drugs from their lives and never miss them.

Speaking in tongues makes me high. It makes me experience an altered state of consciousness. It lets me glimpse another reality — infinite realities — beyond the scope of my "normal" state of consciousness.
— thirty-year-old housewife

Suggested Reading

For all of the talk about alternatives to drugs, precious little is in print on the subject.

The Book of Highs: 250 Methods for Altering Your Consciousness Without Drugs by Edward Rosenfeld (New York:

Quadrangle/New York Times Book Co., 1973) is a unique compilation of practical techniques and further references.

Mind Games: The Guide to Inner Space by Robert Masters and Jean Houston (New York: Viking, 1972) is a manual of exercises in guided fantasy and trance states. The authors have written extensively about psychedelic experiences and are well qualified to discuss altered states of consciousness.

A similar book is *Passages: A Guide for Pilgrims of the Mind* by Marriane S. Andersen and Louis M. Savary (New York: Harper & Row, 1972). Robert S. de Ropp's *The Master Game: Pathways to Higher Consciousness Beyond the Drug Experience* (New York: Delta, 1968) is an excellent book, also intended as a practical guide.

Alternate States of Consciousness edited by Norman E. Zinberg (New York: Free Press, 1977) is a collection of interesting articles by experts in this new field of research; it is more theoretical than practical. Finally, Andrew Weil's *The Marriage of the Sun and Moon: A Quest for Unity in Consciousness* (Boston: Houghton Mifflin, 1980) gives firsthand accounts of various nondrug highs and points out their relationship to drug experiences.

14

Final Words

THE SUBJECT OF DRUGS produces strong emotional reactions in many people, as we have frequently noted. Given that fact, we anticipate that our book will provoke some controversy. The controversy will probably center on the question of whether giving this information to young people will encourage them to try or to use drugs. We would like to address that question head-on.

The truth about drugs cannot do harm. It may offend sensibilities and disturb those who do not want to hear it but it cannot hurt people. On the other hand, false information can and does lead people to hurt themselves and others.

Our intention is not to encourage drug use by anyone, nor is it to discourage drug use. As we wrote at the very beginning, young people (and adults, for that matter) must decide for themselves which drugs, if any, to use and which to reject. We strongly recommend adopting alternatives to drugs whenever possible and we strongly recommend learning to use drugs wisely rather than falling into habits of excess, dependence, and abuse.

People make decisions on the basis of the information available to them. The more accurate the information, the better their decisions will be. We have worked hard to present balanced information that is as accurate as our best efforts can determine. We have not tried to make any drug attractive in our selection of facts.

If we have played down concerns about some drugs — say, the health hazards of marijuana — we have done so because they are products of bias and not in accord with our experience or compatible with the results of good scientific inquiry. In the end, such exaggeration of the dangers of marijuana leads more people to try the drug and more people to abuse it. We have countered those misconceptions by emphasizing what we see as a real danger of marijuana: the ease of sliding into a dependent relationship with it by smoking it unconsciously and excessively.

If we have stressed the ill effects of accepted drugs — say, those of coffee or antihistamines — we have done so because they do accord with good scientific evidence and with our experience, and because we worry that ignorance of these hazards results in widespread overuse with attendant consequences on physical and mental health.

In short, we sincerely believe that the information we have presented in these pages is reliable and will enable people to make intelligent choices about the use of drugs, which should help to prevent drug abuse before it starts.

Permit us to repeat the most important points we have made:

There are no good or bad drugs, only good or bad uses of drugs. Drug abuse is not any use of a disapproved substance; abuse is the use of any substance in ways that impair physical or mental health or social functioning and productivity. Abuse develops from bad relationships with drugs, and learning to recognize such relationships early is one key to preventing abuse. Bad relationships with drugs begin with ignorance or loss of awareness of the nature of a substance and its effects and overuse of it to the point of losing the initial desired effect. Overuse, in turn, leads to difficulty in leaving the drug alone and to eventual impairment of health and productivity.

People must learn to look at and analyze their own and others' relationships with drugs. Because seeing your own behavior for what it is is often difficult, it is worth paying attention to other people's views of your uses of drugs and helpful to tell them your views of their uses of drugs.

Recognizing drug abuse is not a matter of searching a child's room for cigarette papers or looking for dilated eyes or certain styles of dress or types of behavior. It involves the ability to know dependence in oneself and others, to watch how experiences with drugs change over time, to observe changes in health and look for correlations with drug use, to see whether drug habits interfere with work at school or on the job, to see whether they promote associations with undesirable people. This kind of analysis is a lot harder than searching rooms for cigarette papers.

Learning to recognize drug abuse is important, because treatment is not easy, and the earlier a problem comes to light, the better chance there is of correcting it. Prevention of drug abuse is always much easier than treatment. As we have said before, prevention depends on being informed, being aware, and exploring alternatives to drugs. For those who decide to use drugs, prevention depends also on associating with people who use drugs wisely rather than with people who abuse them, and on making intelligent choices about what substances to use and how to use them.

Treatment is another matter. Even with the best help possible, the only alternative for many abusers is to give up their drugs forever and admit they have lost the chance to be in good relationships with those substances. In any case, treatment must begin with an abuser's own recognition that abuse exists and is a problem, and it will depend for its success on an individual's motivation to change. (Alcoholics Anonymous, Overeaters Anonymous, and other such self-help groups take this same position.) A drug abuser who is insufficiently motivated will not be cured by any approach.

Treating drug abuse often requires outside help: from doctors, counselors, clergy, and other professionals trained to advise people in trouble. Deciding where to turn for needed help is rarely easy, since some of the people most eager to work with drug abusers are in no way qualified to do the job. Above all, never put yourself or a child, relative, or friend in treatment for a drug problem with anyone you do not trust or consider fully informed and qualified, no matter what degree or certification the person holds.

Drug-abuse treatment centers are often staffed by ex-addicts. Such counselors may not be the best people to go to for help in improving relationships with drugs, since they failed to form good ones themselves. Many reformed abusers behave like self-righteous fanatics when they appear in public: they inflame discussions about drugs, polarize audiences, and obstruct the drug-education process. It is also worth considering that the drug-abuse treatment profession has a vested interest in seeing drug abuse continue; its members make their living from the problem.

It is uncertain whether going to doctors for help is the best course of action. Medical schools do not teach much about the effects of psychoactive drugs. Unless physicians take the trouble to inform themselves, they are as likely as others to propagate untruths. Doctors have caused a great deal of the drug abuse of the past hundred years by carelessly prescribing opiates, cocaine, amphetamines, and tranquilizers without having clear ideas of the nature of those substances. Also, doctors themselves may be in bad relationships with alcohol, tobacco, coffee, and other stimulants and depressants legally available to them.

In sum, finding reliable help with drug problems is not simple. You have to shop around, ask questions, and use your own judgment. Do not hesitate to ask a prospective counselor to explain to you his or her attitudes toward drugs and recommendations for treatment of abuse. If you agree with the ideas in these pages, you might ask the person to read this book as a basis for your initial discussions.

If all of our warnings and cautions sound discouraging, it is because the treatment of drug abuse is discouraging. For that reason we stress prevention as the better course and come back to solid, truthful information about drugs as the single best measure.

Suggested Reading lists follow most chapters, and we urge you to use them as a guide if you require more detail on a particular subject. The more you inform yourself on the complicated and ever-present issue of drugs, the more you can protect yourself and those around you from trouble, and the more you will be doing your part to steer society onto a less destructive course.

Appendix: First-Person Accounts
and Comments

Glossary

Index

First-Person Accounts and Comments

Drugs in High School

A lot of kids in my high school were into drugs. The upperclassmen — myself included — smoked pot regularly and drank (mostly beer) on the weekends. The big status drug was cocaine, only no one could ever afford it. There was one kid who used to steal it from his parents, though, a little every day, and save it up for parties.

The main reason most kids took drugs — in my opinion — was peer pressure. Of course, we didn't admit that to ourselves. We weren't even conscious of it, really. It wasn't too obvious; if it had been obvious it probably would have been a lot easier to resist. But it was a subtle thing, an attitude. We didn't think about it, but it was there.

— twenty-year-old man, college sophomore

The Coffee Cantata

Johann Sebastian Bach (1685–1750) wrote the Coffee Cantata around 1732, when the new drink began to leave the male society of coffee houses in Germany and invade private homes, where ladies began to consume it. In the cantata, the father is angry because his daughter is a coffee addict. He threatens not to provide her with a husband unless she promises to stop drinking it. Here are a few excerpts from their dialogue:

FATHER: O wicked child! Ungrateful daughter, why will you not respect my wishes and cease this coffee drinking?

DAUGHTER: Dear Father, be not so unkind; I love my cup of coffee at least three times a day, and if this pleasure you deny me, what else on earth is there to live for?

DAUGHTER [continues in solo aria]:   Far beyond all other pleasures, rarer than jewels or treasures, sweeter than grape from the vine. Yes! Yes! Greatest of pleasures! Coffee, coffee, how I love its flavor, and if you would win my favor, yes! Yes! let me have coffee, let me have my coffee strong.

FATHER: Well, pretty daughter, you must choose. If sense of duty you have none, then I must try another way. My patience is well nigh exhausted! Now listen! From your dress allowance I will take one half. Your next birthday should soon be here; no present will you get from me.

DAUGHTER: . . . how cruel! But I will forgive you and consolation find in coffee . . .

* * *

FATHER: Now, hearken to my last word. If coffee you must have, then a husband you shall not have.

DAUGHTER: O father! O horror! Not a husband?

FATHER: I swear it, and I mean it too.

DAUGHTER: O harsh decree! O cruel choice, between a husband and my joy. I'll strive no more; my coffee I surrender.

FATHER: At last you have regained your senses.

[The daughter sings a melancholy aria of resignation.]

TENOR: And now, behold the happy father as forth he goes in search of a husband, rich and handsome, for his daughter. But the crafty little maiden has quite made up her mind, that, ere she gives consent to marriage, her lover must make a solemn promise that she may have her coffee whenever and wherever she pleases.

Coffee Has Never Failed Me

In the morning I drink two cups of coffee. If I don't, I feel irritable. If I drink three cups, I get a little speedy, but with two I feel just about right.

If I drink coffee after about three in the afternoon, I cannot fall asleep when I like to, about eleven-thirty. If I drink coffee after dinner, as little as a half cup, I lie awake long past midnight. If I have something important or risky to do the next day, especially some public performance, coffee late in the day invariably interacts with my nervousness to produce stark insomnia.

This sleeplessness after coffee feels pharmacological. I can reach a dreamy peacefulness and experience some of the floating state that usually precedes sleep for me, but then I just hang on the edge, never quite slipping into unconsciousness. When I get up the next morning (angry at myself for not having slept), I feel relaxed but not rested by my seven hours in bed.

When I know that I have a long drive ahead of me, one that will mean driving late into the night or straight through it, I don't drink coffee for two or three days before. (I settle for lower doses of caffeine in tea or cola.) On the night of the drive I drink coffee twice, first a cup or two when I get drowsy at my usual bedtime, then two cups or more about three hours later. If I have been drinking coffee steadily for the few days before, I seem to get less stimulant effect from drinking it at night. It is almost a matter of "saving up" the coffee I would have consumed on the two or three days preceding and then drinking it on a particular night to keep me awake on the road. Used in this way, coffee has been a great help to me and has never failed me.

— thirty-nine-year-old man, college administrator

Coffee Addiction

My wife and I have drunk a lot of coffee for many years. I used to be a cigarette smoker but stopped with great difficulty twelve years ago; she still smokes, and I don't think she will ever be able to stop. I begin the day with two cups of coffee and drink about six more cups until din-nertime. Recently we started drinking decaffeinated coffee with dinner, because we found the regular kind made it hard for us to fall asleep at bedtime.

A few years ago I developed a shake in my left hand. The doctors call it a tremor and have no explanation or treatment for it. In the past year it got worse and made me self-conscious. A number of people told me that caffeine might be causing it or, at least, making it worse, so I thought it would be a good idea to cut it out. Since I never thought that coffee did much for me or was much of a drug, I never thought it would be hard for me to stop.

My wife also thought of coffee as just a pleasant drink that we liked, and she agreed that we should switch to decaffeinated com-pletely. So we did. I didn't notice any difference the first day, but on the second day I got very tired at my office and started to get a bad head-ache. I decided to come home early. When I arrived, I found my wife lying on the couch groaning. She said she had one of the worst head-aches of her life and couldn't even stand up. Since my headache was steadily getting worse, I realized we must be experiencing a reaction to lack of caffeine. I told my wife that, but she refused to believe me. I told her I would prove it. I went to the kitchen and fixed us both cups of strong regular coffee. Within ten minutes of drinking them, we both felt our headaches disappear as if by magic and felt like our old selves. It astonished me to see how addicted we were to caffeine; my wife could scarcely believe it, since she was even less aware than I that coffee can be an addicting drug.

Since then we have been trying to wean ourselves off caffeine by gradually substituting decaffeinated coffee for regular. We've cut our consumption in half so far but still cannot do without the two cups in the morning, even after a year of trying. We're determined to do it, however, and I know we'll succeed. Seeing the addiction for what it was gave us the motivation we needed.

— sixty-eight-year-old man, lawyer

Kicking the Chocolate Habit

Five years ago, hoping to kick a chocolate habit that was significantly affecting my life, I enrolled in a program at the Shick Center for the Control of Smoking, Alcoholism, and Overeating, in Los Angeles. I was then thirty-three. I could not remember the last time I had managed to get through a whole day without eating chocolate in one form or another, usually in quantities most people would regard as excessive, if not appalling.

Though not overweight, I indulged many of my chocolate cravings in secret, often in the middle of the night, when, if I had no chocolate in the house, I would think nothing of getting in my car and driving halfway across L.A. to an all-night supermarket for a fix. Although the Shick people told me they could cure my chocolate addiction in ten sessions, I was skeptical. My behavior was so compulsive and out of control that the best I thought I could hope for was a slight, temporary reduction of the cravings I suffered constantly. Still, I was willing to try anything.

The Shick Center places no importance on will power, since it believes any form of self-imposed denial is doomed to failure. Instead, it uses a behavior-modification technique so simple as to seem ludicrous. Following instructions, I arrived for my first session with plenty of my favorite food (Hershey bars) and was seated in front of a mirror and handed a paper plate. A gadget was then strapped to my wrist that could give a very low-level electric shock. Far from being painful, this sensation was barely noticeable. I was told it was meant to have a purely subliminal effect. Thus equipped, I spent the next half-hour chewing mouthfuls of chocolate, which, instead of swallowing, I had to spit out onto the paper plate, all the while watching myself in the mirror.

During this first session, my skepticism hardened into utter disbelief. The mild revulsion I felt at the sight of seeing myself spit out the chocolate was more than offset by the pleasure of having it in my mouth. I couldn't see how such an absurd procedure could even scratch the surface of a problem as profound as mine, and were it not for the program's money-back guarantee, I would have dropped out then and there.

The following six sessions were carbon copies of the first. Toward the end of my seventh visit, I remember thinking, "This can't possibly be working; I still love the taste of chocolate as much as ever." Meanwhile, the program made no attempt to restrict what I ate on my own, and my chocolate consumption continued unabated.

It was not until the eighth session that I experienced a trace — it was the merest inkling — of something changing. It wasn't that I liked the taste of chocolate any less, but somehow I did not feel quite so compelled to put it in my mouth. Then, midway through the ninth session, I sensed a subtle but definite change. I didn't experience anything like distaste, but somehow eating the chocolate became automatic and without pleasure. I was still doubtful, especially about lasting effects, but the change was a revelation.

Preposterous as it may sound, I walked out of the tenth session completely cured. Although chocolate does not disgust me, I have no desire to eat it, ever. Flavors I never cared for before — vanilla, for example, or strawberry — appeal much more to me now, and I will choose them over chocolate every time. I don't consciously avoid chocolate out of fear of getting hooked again, either. I suppose I could get hooked again if I worked at it, but even though I test myself occasionally, my indifference to it remains the same.

Frankly, I am mystified by what happened and to this day cannot explain it. Being addicted to chocolate was so much a part of my definition of myself that it constantly amazes me to think that I am free of it. Needless to say, I am very grateful. The only problem is, I am now addicted (though somewhat less severely) to cake . . .

— thirty-eight-year-old woman, social worker

Trouble with Cocaine

I first tried cocaine when I was twenty-three. I had been using speed to help me with schoolwork and with my art. Cocaine was much more expensive than speed in those days and seemed less powerful, but I began to read a lot of information about the dangers of speed and thought cocaine might not be as harmful.

A few years later I sold cocaine for a short time, although I still was not very involved with it. When I went to Europe on a vacation, I gave away what I had.

About 1970, when I was twenty-eight, cocaine was more common, partly because the drug generation was older and had more money and partly because the dangers of speed were then well known. I found that coke gave me a good boost for getting work done. When I snorted it, I would feel inspired, brilliant, and energized. My art work went much faster with it because I could really focus on it and feel good at the same time. The ideas I got on coke were good ones, and I could get them down on paper. I came to see cocaine as an inducement and reward for getting work done.

Four years later I began to realize that I could not work easily without cocaine. If I didn't use it, I felt bored, tired, and out of focus, which made me want to have it around all the time. As a result I spent more and more money on it. I think I also began to get less patient, more critical, and paranoid. I started selling coke to friends to cover my needs, although I found dealing with friends as customers confusing and stressful. I got more and more difficult to be around. I was under a lot of work pressure, too, having to renovate a house I had acquired. I felt the need to rely on coke more and more to squeeze creative energy out of myself.

In 1978 — I was thirty-six then — a number of personal problems built up to an emotional crisis. A long-term love relationship broke up, and I ran into a dry spell with my art. I turned even more to coke to sustain me during this period. At first a gram might last me a week, but soon I was using half a gram to a gram every day, sometimes having the first snort as soon as I got up. I would go for days without sleep. Also, I paid little attention to my diet. At one point, I had to go to the hospital with severe pain that turned out to be a kidney stone. I think it resulted from episodes of bad dehydration, since coke made me urinate more, but I would put off getting something to drink for hours while I buried myself in work.

In order to relax while using cocaine so heavily, I had to drink alcohol or take Valium. Even so I would often lie in bed for hours with my heart racing, unable to fall asleep. I was really living in the extremes — either groggy and depressed or speeding. Finally, all that coke made me crazy. It gave me false inspiration and a kind of tunnel vision that hurt my creative efforts. Also, I began to suffer severe depressions. I'd play hide-and-seek games with the coke, locking it away and telling myself I wouldn't use it today. But as long as I knew it was there, I couldn't stop thinking about it and finally would give in and use it. Then I'd feel guilty as well.

I finally stopped taking it because the depressions outweighed the highs. After a few months I tried it again but got the same results: depression and no high. I haven't used cocaine since then — it's been over a year now. I still miss it and have had to relearn how to work without it. I feel strongly that I have to avoid any contact with that drug from now on.

— thirty-nine-year-old man, artist

Speeding Through European History

I was miserable and homesick during my first year at college and, as a result, wasn't a particularly good student. In fact, I spent the better part of my time bad-mouthing the school and sitting around feeling sorry for myself, and very little time studying. Therefore, when midterms came around I had little hope of distinguishing myself. I decided to try and make up for lost time by staying up all night to study for my European history exam, but by midnight the text was blurring before my eyes. I was studying in the dining room of my dorm with several other girls. Seeing me losing my struggle to stay awake, an upperclassman took pity on me and offered me a green-and-white capsule along with the promise that my drowsiness would be cured by taking it. I took it without a second thought, and within half an hour or so found myself studying like mad. Not only was I completely engrossed in European history, I felt exhilarated; I was actually enjoying myself for the first time in months.

You always hear stories about people taking exams on amphetamines and thinking they've done brilliantly only to find out later that they wrote page after page of incomprehensible gibberish. I almost wish that had happened in my case. I got an A on my history exam — as I was sure I had — and have been involved, to some extent, with amphetamines ever since.

— forty-two-year-old woman, writer

A College Speed Freak

I was a speed freak in college but did not know it, because a doctor got me to take it and never told me I could get hooked. I was about thirty pounds overweight and had never been able to diet for long. A school doctor started me on daily doses of Desoxyn and told me it would suppress my appetite. It did. It also made me feel great, at least at first. He also gave me a diet to follow, and I soon lost most of my excess weight. After several months, however, I began getting irritable and depressed and also didn't sleep well. I ate more when I was in these moods and gained some weight back. I found that taking more Desoxyn made me feel better and eat less.

It never occurred to me that the Desoxyn could affect my mood. I was completely ignorant of what it was; I think I considered it a kind of dietary supplement that took away hunger. My doctor never made me feel I needed to worry about taking it all the time. Soon I was taking three times the original dose.

Even when speed began to get a bad reputation in the late 1960s I didn't know I was on it. I was really shocked to learn that Desoxyn was just a brand name for methamphetamine and even more shocked to find that I couldn't stop taking it. If I tried to cut down the dose or stop, I would be groggy, depressed, and unable to concentrate or do my schoolwork. I would also eat a lot and gain weight. By the way, I also drank a lot of coffee and smoked cigarettes, so I was really a heavy user of stimulants.

When I told the doctor I was worried about being addicted, he made light of my fears, saying Desoxyn was a safe drug. It took many visits over the next year to convince him that I had a drug problem and took me another year beyond that to get off speed entirely. When I did, I was back where I started as far as being overweight. I feel I was a victim of that doctor's ignorance and probably of the drug company's promotion of the stuff for weight loss. Also, I know I was not an unusual case, because I have met other people who had similar experiences. I do not think I will ever take any kind of amphetamine again, because I am afraid that I would easily fall back into the same pattern of addictive use. Maybe those drugs have some good uses, but not in the way I took them.

— thirty-nine-year-old man, lawyer

Speed in College: Another View

As a college student in the 1960s I used speed to take important exams. Caffeine never helped me stay up; I could drink all the coffee I could stand or take many times the recommended dose of No-Doz and still fall asleep. So I went to the student health services, where a doctor listened to my story of getting sleepy when I had to study. He gave me a prescription for Dexamyl. The first time I took the stuff I felt so good that I wrote a paper for a course effortlessly. I took another capsule the next day and got about half the effect. That made me realize I should not use it regularly.

The pattern I developed was to save the speed for the day of a big morning exam. I'd stay up studying as late as I could — say till 3 A.M. — then go to sleep and set the alarm for seven. When I woke up, I'd study a little more and take a Dexamyl capsule when I left my room to walk to the exam. By the time I got the questions I'd be buzzing with energy and confidence and be eager to start writing.

I did well in all the exams I took that way and never got any complaints that I'd written my name over and over. For me Dexamyl really increased concentration and mental performance. (Of course, I had to know the material; it didn't put information in my head if I did not study.)

After I had made several visits to the student health service for new prescriptions, the doctor gave me an unlimited one that I used for several years and enabled me to give Dexamyl to classmates who also needed it at exam time. I never used speed in any other situations, and no one I knew in college had problems with it. I suppose that kind of prescription is not allowed anymore, and I know amphetamines have a bad reputation today, but I think we used them sensibly, and they helped us cope with a system that paralyzed many students with anxiety.

— thirty-nine-year-old man, writer

A Nonaddicted Smoker

Like Mark Twain, I find it easy to give up smoking; I have done it countless times. In fact, I consider myself a nonaddicted smoker, since I have been smoking cigarettes on and off for twenty-five years without ever getting so hooked I couldn't stop just like *that* whenever I chose to. I would see nothing extraordinary about this, were it not for the wonder and admiration it excites in other people. Since it is mostly unheard of to smoke cigarettes only now and then, acquaintances regard me as a woman of superhuman will power, a notion I hate to disabuse them of.

However, the sad truth is, I have no more will power than anyone else and probably less than many. What saves me from being a cigarette junkie is that I recognized early how easy it would be for me to get hooked on tobacco, and, knowing that if I did get hooked I'd hate myself, I have always been very careful to keep my smoking under control.

For one thing, I never smoke before five o'clock in the afternoon. That, in itself, might seem adequate insurance against addiction, but, even though I have no desire for a cigarette before that time, I have been known to smoke up to five in a row once I begin — making myself very sick in the process. So I limit myself to one cigarette before dinner and try not to smoke more than five or six in the course of an evening. Also, I monitor my consumption very closely, and whenever I notice a rising trend, I swear off entirely for a few days.

Since my husband is a confirmed and heavy smoker, it requires some effort on my part to refrain entirely for days at a time. On the other hand, having him around helps me in the long run because he provides a living example of the sort of dependency I want so much to avoid.

— thirty-seven-year-old woman, housewife

Love versus Cigarettes

These days I run into lots of people who have stopped smoking, and they always say, "You could do it, too." I suppose they're right in theory. I mean, in theory I could run the triathalon if I put my mind to it, but in practice I know it isn't so.

I come from a long line of smokers. At seventy my mother still smokes heavily. Her mother smoked well into her eighties (and lived to be ninety-three). I took up the habit at age thirteen, and for the next twenty years I never once seriously considered denying myself the pleasure smoking afforded me.

Then, several years ago, I fell madly in love with an ex-smoker, a man who, though broad-minded in other respects, was a fanatic on the subject of cigarettes. He forbade smoking anywhere in his vicinity — not only in his own house and car but also in other people's houses and cars, as well as in restaurants and movie theaters, where he would not hesitate to browbeat people into putting out their cigarettes even when they were legally within their rights to smoke.

Very early in our relationship, I realized it would be futile to expect him to compromise on this issue. Not only did he object to cigarette smoke in the air he breathed, he hated the smell of it on my breath, in my hair or clothing. He was also highly sensitive to the odor of cigarettes, and though I bent over backwards to avoid offending him, my efforts were mostly unsuccessful. I grew increasingly defensive and insecure, and soon had to face the fact that we couldn't possibly have a long-term, intimate relationship unless I quit smoking. I therefore resolved to do so, and one day, feeling very virtuous, I tossed out my cigarettes and went cold turkey.

My friend assured me that I would soon begin to feel great as a result of not smoking, but in fact the discomfort I experienced from abstinence was intense and unrelenting, even after five weeks. Smoking had become so woven into the fabric of my life that everything seemed to come unraveled without it. I could not get my mind off cigarettes for more than ten seconds at a time. I craved them not only every minute of every day but also in my dreams at night.

Naturally, my agony put a lot of stress on what was still an untried and untested relationship, and the relationship did not bear up well under it, I'm afraid. No doubt I wanted much more credit and consideration from my friend than I deserved, but I also deserved, I think, somewhat more than I got. Having gone through the ordeal himself, he was, if anything, less compassionate. He did not want to hear about my suffering and put me down for continuing to make such a fuss. Then, after five weeks of steadily mounting tension, he had to go to Europe on business for a month. I started smoking again as soon as his plane took off.

When my friend returned from Europe, he was most unhappy to find that instead of being out of the woods I was right back at square one. He was willing to try again, but this time, instead of urging me to quit for reasons of my own health and well-being, he wanted me to do it for him. What meant more to me — him or cigarettes? That was the choice I was faced with. In other words, it was a test.

Well, to make a long story short, I failed the test — not once or twice, but repeatedly, almost every day for ten straight months, in fact. Had my lapses been matters merely between me and my conscience, they would have been bad enough. But, as I said, my friend was very sensitive to the odor of tobacco. No matter what precautions I took, he was able, even hours after the fact, to smell the evidence on my breath. So I was constantly humiliated as well, and my failures became the subject of endless arguments, and, toward the end of the affair, the cause of several knockdown, drag-out fights. There were, of course, other differences between us, but the issue of smoking became a sort of lightning rod, attracting more and more of the emotional charge.

I had always thought I'd be able to kick my addiction for someone I loved. That assumption turned out to be wrong. In the end, when forced to choose between love and cigarettes, I chose cigarettes. It was that simple.

I did make one resolution at the time, which I have stuck to ever since. It was that I would never again become involved with a man who does not smoke cigarettes.

— forty-one-year-old woman, teacher

I Like Alcohol

I like alcohol. It is a powerful drug and, God knows, for some people a hellish one, but if used carefully it can give great pleasure. After a long, hard day, the splendid warm glow that strong drink provides is one of my favorite feelings; it starts in the pit of my stomach, then spreads to my limbs and brain. I know that alcohol is a depressant, but it acts and feels like a gentle relaxant — of the spirit as well as of the physical body. Just notice the increased vivacity and noise level at a cocktail party after a drink has been served to see how alcohol can put people at ease emotionally.

Aside from the pleasureful intoxication of strong drink, I also enjoy the tastes of lighter forms of alcohol. Few sensations are more delightful than the wet but dry taste of cold beer to a parched throat. The subtle, taste-enhancing, enriching relationship of wine to food is a subject that has inspired many poets and writers far more capable than I of putting words together, but I can tell you that what they say is true. The fascinating, complex flavor of good wine can be profoundly sensual.

— sixty-two-year-old man, psychoanalyst

Bad Drinking Habits

I was sixteen when I first got drunk. It was a revelation, more fun than a barrel of monkeys. I screamed and hollered and carried on and did somersaults and hugged my friends (who were also drunk) and just had a blast. Naturally, I kept wanting to repeat the experience.

Pretty soon a group of my high-school friends and I got into regular weekend parties where we'd get drunk (usually on hard liquor) and lose our inhibitions. Sometimes we'd even bring a bottle to school and sneak out between classes to drink a little. No one knew anything about pot or other drugs in those days. Alcohol was it. It was our main way of getting high and so was very important to us.

When I went away to college, I continued my pattern of using alcohol to get high, mostly at weekend parties. But two things began to happen that bothered me. First, from doing it over and over, the alcohol high lost a little of its fascination for me. Although I still liked it, it didn't measure up to those early experiences in high school. Secondly, I started getting bad hangovers. I mean I'd really be sick as a dog the next day, and I didn't like that at all. The price seemed much too high to pay for a few hours of fun.

I used to tell myself I'd only drink to the point of getting pleasantly high, but every single time I'd go beyond it. Before I'd know it, I'd be stumbling around, being loud and jovial, insensitive to pain. I'd feel great at the time, and I'd also know what was in store for me. Usually, the sick effects would start when I'd try to go to sleep drunk: terrible nausea with the room spinning. Every serious drinker knows that one. And the next day I'd be totally out of action, feeling as if I'd been poisoned, which I guess I had. I got really scared one time when I woke up like that and couldn't remember anything of the night before.

Although I kept trying to use alcohol moderately, whenever I'd set out to get high on it, I would always keep on drinking till I got drunk, no matter how many resolutions I made not to.

About that time, pot came along. It took me a little while to learn to get high on it, but when I did, it seemed much better than alcohol for me. There was no problem of taking too much and behaving badly, no getting sick, and no hangover. Becoming a pot smoker got me out of my bad drinking habits. I think if I'd kept them up, I would now be in real trouble.

I've tried various drugs since those days and don't think anything comes close to alcohol in terms of raw strength and potential for trouble. I couldn't learn to control it well, and I see many people around me who have the same problem.

— thirty-seven-year-old man, college professor

An Overdose of Downers

The old saying "The cobbler's children go without shoes" applies to the children of physicians, too. Because they deal with sick people all day long, doctors tend to give short shrift to the complaints of family members. As the daughter of a medical doctor, I should know. When I or any of my brothers or sisters came down with anything more serious than a hangnail, my father's standard procedure was to ply us with sleeping pills.

When I was very young, his prescription was for a half grain or so of phenobarbital, but by the time I was in junior high school, whenever I had a sore throat or stuffy nose, I was sent to bed with two Seconals or Nembutals as a matter of course. The theory behind this treatment was that a good night's sleep would cure just about anything, and though it did not always work out that way, I never doubted the basic principle or questioned the wisdom of using drugs to implement it.

Later, when I was living on my own, my father gave me an assortment of sleeping pills to have on hand just in case. Falling asleep was never one of my problems, so I never resorted to them on my own. Then, one night when I had come down with a severe cold, my father stopped by and advised me to take some sedatives to be sure to get a good night's sleep. I said okay, produced the grab bag of pills, and asked him which to take. He chose two of the biggest gelatin capsules I had ever seen. They were Placidyl, he told me, 250 milligrams each. I protested, sure that one would more than do the job, but he insisted they were very mild, and that 500 milligrams was the standard dose. After I'd taken them, he left.

Meanwhile, I had been waiting for a neighbor to come and walk my dog in the park across the street. After twenty minutes or so, when she still hadn't arrived, I decided I'd take the dog out quickly myself. I was starting to feel groggy and wanted to go to sleep.

I lost consciousness almost as soon as I reached the street. All of a sudden there was a fantastic explosion of lights, and I remember looking up at the sky, exclaiming "Wow!" before blacking out. That must have been around ten-thirty. When I came to, it was after midnight, and people were shaking me and slapping my face. I was in the park, where some other dog walkers had discovered me on a bench in a stupor. Apparently, the dog had dragged me in a somnambulent state all the way up the block, across a big street, and into the park. The people who found me had been slapping me for several minutes without success. Figuring I had either overdosed on something accidentally or made a suicide attempt, they were on the verge of calling an ambulance. It was obvious to everyone that I was heavily drugged, and, of course, they were all upset. When I realized what had happened, I was beside myself with rage.

Calling my father on the telephone to rant and rave brought no satisfaction. He not only refused to accept any responsibility for what had occurred — sticking to his story about 500 milligrams of Placidyl being a mild dose — he even tried to shift the blame onto me by suggesting that I had some deep, unconscious motive for passing out in the street. I hung up, consciously motivated to strangle him.

As it turned out, my father had given me not 500 milligrams of Placidyl but twice that amount: 1000 milligrams, or, as the package insert put it, enough to knock out a woman in labor. Nevertheless, he continued to make light of the incident and deny any negligence on his part.

On the whole, the experience was very valuable for me because it taught me something people need to know — namely, that it is good to be skeptical about doctors (whether or not they are relatives) and the casual ways they dispense drugs.

— thirty-eight-year-old woman, artist

Experiences with Quaalude

Many of my friends and I began using methaqualone, or Quaaludes, in the 1960s. We take them on occasion only and like the way they remove inhibitions and ease social interactions. I know a lot of folks who consider Quaalude their drug of choice, especially for having fun and partying.

I've seen Quaalude produce hilarious situations. One time I went with a group of friends to dinner at a fancy Italian restaurant. Most of us took Quaalude before leaving the house. We ordered dinner in high spirits, and when it came started eating. Just then, one woman who had taken a double dose passed out and fell face first into her plate of spaghetti. Everyone else stood up and applauded.

I've also seen Quaalude lead to tragic situations. Everyone knows that downers and driving don't mix. I know a woman who was trying to cope with severe depression by taking Quaalude. One night, after exceeding her usual dosage, she went out and almost lost her life in an auto accident. She ran into a parked car.

I've seen other people become violent on Quaalude, then not remember it afterwards — just as with alcohol. One man who saw me professionally told me he once took three Quaaludes and went to bed. The next thing he remembered was being awakened about two hours later by his frightened wife, who told him he had been beating her.

There is no question that Quaalude can be dangerous when used irresponsibly, or that it can be addicting. As a recreational drug, taken on occasion in a responsible manner, it seems to me safe and interesting and gives me an experience different from anything else.

One of the rules I follow is to know my tolerance so that I take the right dose. Black-market Quaaludes are more of a problem, because their quality is uncertain. Usually they contain less methaqualone than pharmaceutical Quaaludes, but they really vary. I've seen two people with equal tolerance each take one black-market Quaalude and experience different effects. So knowing your drug is important, too.

The other rules that are most important are not to mix Quaalude with alcohol and not to mix Quaalude with driving.

— thirty-six-year-old man, drug counselor

Down on Valium

I hope I never hear of Valium again. A university physician gave it to me as a "muscle relaxant" when I had a pinched nerve in my neck that caused muscle spasms in my right shoulder and weakness in my right hand. He did not tell me anything about the mental effects of Valium, so I was quite unprepared for them. All I remember of the next few days is that I could not concentrate in my office. Then my secretary and wife began acting strange. Only when I stopped taking the drug did I realize how bizarre my behavior had become while I was on it. I would stare blankly into space when people talked to me, not remember anything said to me, and be unable to think or reason. Also, I had no sense that anything was wrong. I think Valium turned me into a kind of zombie for those few days. I can't understand why anyone would want to take it.

— sixty-two-year-old man, university professor

Valium as a Tool

I first began taking Valium ten years ago to relieve anxiety and very quickly came to depend on it for writing, or, more exactly, for beginning to write. Once I am at my desk and have actually begun to work, I am fine; the problem for me is to get there in the first place. What I discovered was that very soon after I took a dose of Valium, I felt high, and that during the brief period that the high lasted, getting to my desk was a whole lot easier.

By now, after ten years of experimenting, I have learned that like any tool, Valium has its limitations. It works best on an empty stomach, for example, and when it comes to dosage, less is definitely more. Two and a half milligrams is the right dose for me; more than that makes me feel groggy. Also, since I become tolerant to its effects if I take it more than two days running, I have to use it intermittently.

Even when I observe all the rules and take Valium under ideal conditions, the period of grace it affords me is extremely brief. Once its effects begin to come on, I have about fifteen minutes in which to capitalize on them. During that critical period, if I happen to be distracted by a phone call or a neighbor dropping by, all is lost. That sounds hard to believe, I know, but it has happened to me many times, and whenever it does, that's it: the day is shot. Besides being too anxious to get to my desk, I will be furious — positively fit to be tied.

— thirty-nine-year-old woman, writer

An Anesthetic Revelation

I once inhaled a pretty full dose of ether, with the determination to put on record, at the earliest moment of regaining consciousness, the thought I should find uppermost in my mind. The mighty music of the triumphal march into nothingness reverberated through my brain, and filled me with a sense of infinite possibilities, which made me an archangel for a moment. The veil of eternity was lifted. The one great truth which underlies all human experience and is the key to all the mysteries that philosophy has sought in vain to solve, flashed upon me in a sudden revelation. Henceforth all was clear: a few words had lifted my intelligence to the level of the knowledge of the cherubim. As my natural condition returned, I remembered my resolution; and, staggering to my desk, I wrote, in ill-shaped, straggling characters, the all-embracing truth still glimmering in my consciousness. The words were these (children may smile; the wise will ponder): "A strong smell of turpentine prevails throughout."

> — Oliver Wendell Holmes (1809–1894),
> American physician and author,
> from a lecture given in 1870

The Need for Opiates

The first opiate I ever took was codeine. I snorted it. It made me feel right for the first time in my life. I said to myself, "Aha, this is what I've been missing." I never felt right from as far back as I can remember, and I was always trying different ways to change how I felt. I used lots of drugs, including pot, downers, tranquilizers, and alcohol, but none of them ever really did it for me. Codeine was a revelation, and I've been an opiate user ever since.

That first time I was twenty-three. Before long I was addicted, although I've always snorted dope, never shot it. Opiates have caused me lots of trouble, but what they do for my head is worth it. Now I'm thirty-four and am on methadone maintenance. I don't think methadone is the best opiate for me; it makes me sweat terribly and has some other effects on my body I don't like, but it's great to be able to get what I need legally, so that I can spend time on things other than scoring. I hope one day more people will realize that some of us have to have opiates just to feel normal.

> — thirty-four-year-old woman, rock singer

Opiate Addiction

I started using heroin in high school, chipped for a long time, then finally became an addict. Presently, I'm on methadone, which works well for me. I use narcotics to keep from feeling sick (withdrawal), to relieve stress, and sometimes for fun. I like to mainline because it's the most economical way to take opiates: heroin is at least three times as active intravenously as orally, although the effects last longer if you take it by mouth.

I've read a lot about opiate users seeking a "rush" by injecting heroin. To me the rush has never been that important. It feels like a pleasant warm feeling, especially in the pit of the stomach, accompanied by deep physical and mental relaxation. (Incidentally, smoking many opiates gives a stronger rush than mainlining, but it is wasteful, because some of the drug is destroyed by heat.) In my experience, chippers are more interested in rushes than addicts. They tend to take narcotics on occasion for fun, whereas addicts take them regularly in order to make it through a troubled world. Regular doses of heroin just make many addicts feel normal; they do not give noticeable rushes.

For me, the rush is secondary to the tranquilizing and pain-relieving effects of opiates. I feel I have a metabolic problem due to lack of endogenous opiatelike drugs. By substituting external narcotics for internal ones, I have probably shut off my body's production of the endogenous substances, and now I have to take opiates regularly to make life bearable. Sometimes, I'll take a higher than usual dose for pleasure and savor the rush, but that's unusual. Oral methadone does not give a rush, and if rushes were so important to addicts, methadone maintenance would not be accepted by so many of them. As I've said, it works for me.

By the way, my health has been generally good since I've been an opiate addict. I don't get colds when other people do, and when I travel in Mexico, I don't get dysentery, although my nonusing companions do, and we eat the same food.

— thirty-year-old man, chemist

LSD and Psilocybin

I have been unable to identify any sign at all of addiction, organic injury, or other, in some way unpleasant aftereffects . . . In my opinion, however, LSD and psilocybin cannot and should not become "pleasure drugs" for the general public. Their effects are such that they lead one beyond the customary (and constraining) coordinate system of space and time, and afford insights into the heaven and hell of one's own self — which can be dangerous to one who is not cut out for that, and hence is not prepared.

According to my experience, only several repeated experiments afford a serious appraisal. I also believe that at least one of these experiments should be undertaken in familiar surroundings (under discreet supervision of a trusted person) and with higher doses. *Only* then might the drug show us its, and our, deepest secret.

— Rudolf Gelpke,
a Swiss professor of Islamic studies
who took LSD and psilocybin
a number of times in 1961

A DMT Disaster

The only time I ever took a psychedelic was a disaster. It was in the early 1960s, and the drug was DMT. I knew nothing about it. Some friends invited me to their place and told me they wanted to share a pleasant experience with me. They said they would inject a small amount of a new drug into my leg. It was safe and would give me a nice feeling for a short time. I agreed to try it.

Within a few minutes of the injection, I was swept into a nightmare world of horrible visions, such as finding myself wading into an ocean where all sorts of monsters attacked me. The real world disappeared so completely I thought I'd never see it again. Even years later I can still recall the feeling of slimy tentacles grabbing my legs and trying to pull me underwater. When I came back from this frightening place, I was so shaken that I stayed in my room for two days. It took me a very long time to get over being afraid of the ocean afterwards, and to this day I have been unable to try another psychedelic, although I am curious about the good effects people have described to me. I think those friends who gave me DMT were not malicious, just irresponsible. I wonder how many others have had similar bad experiences from taking psychedelic drugs with no preparation?

— thirty-five-year-old man, movie producer

Peyote Visions

My first vivid show of mescal colour effects came quickly. I saw the stars, and then, of a sudden, here and there delicate floating films of colour — usually delightful neutral purples and pinks. These came and went — now here, now there. Then an abrupt rush of countless points of white light swept across the field of view, as if the unseen millions of the Milky Way were to flow a sparkling river before the eye. In a minute this was over and the field was dark. Then I began to see zigzag lines of very bright colours . . .

When I opened my eyes all was gone at once. Closing them I began after a long interval to see for the first time definite objects associated with colours. The stars sparkled and passed away. A white spear of grey stone grew up to a huge height, and became a tall, richly finished Gothic tower of very elaborate and definite design, with many rather worn statues standing in the doorways or on stone brackets. As I gazed, every projecting angle, cornice, and even the faces of the stones at their joinings were by degrees covered or hung with clusters of what seemed to be huge precious stones, but uncut, some being more like masses of transparent fruit. These were green, purple, red, and orange; never clear yellow and never blue. All seemed to possess an interior light, and to give the faintest idea of the perfectly satisfying intensity and purity of these gorgeous colour-fruits is quite beyond my power. All the colours I have ever beheld are dull as compared to these.

— from an essay
by Dr. S. Weir Mitchell (1829–1914),
an American physician and novelist
who drank an extract of peyote in 1896

Psychedelic Therapy

As a clinical psychologist who has treated hundreds of patients with psychedelic drugs over the past twenty-five years, I consider LSD, MDA, magic mushrooms, mescaline, and the rest to be the most valuable therapeutic tools I know to show people how they can change in positive directions.

Because my use of these drugs is not approved under current laws or standards of practice, I cannot publish my findings or engage openly in psychedelic therapy. Still, I have trained many other psychiatrists and psychologists to use this method and have been able to treat many patients successfully. I am very careful in selecting patients for this kind of treatment, very careful in preparing them for a psychedelic session, in conducting the session, and in following it up with the kind of work that enables patients to make practical use of the insights they gain.

Conventional forms of psychotherapy often enable people to understand how their habits of thinking about themselves and others produce frustration and pain, but you can spend years in therapy gaining all this insight and keep on being the same frustrated, neurotic person. One good psychedelic session can make you *feel* what you are doing and show you how to do it differently. In the right hands and settings these drugs can convince you that the worst problem in your life can be solved by changing your own attitudes and ways of perceiving and can motivate you to make the necessary changes.

It is a shame that more doctors and patients do not take advantage of this potential.

— seventy-year-old man, psychologist

Quitting Pot

I smoked marijuana for about seven years, mostly during college and law school. It was great for me at first, a real relaxer and sense-enhancer, and I had a lot of good times with it. Occasionally I had bad reactions to it — paranoia, shaking, pounding heartbeat, and feeling cold all over. Sometimes I'd have this reaction every time I'd smoke over a period of a week or so, then I wouldn't have it again for many months. I don't know what it came from, maybe being in uncomfortable environments or around people I didn't like.

Eventually I became a daily pot smoker, sometimes starting in the morning. It was my main way of relating to other people. However, I started getting less and less effect from it that I liked. In fact, it began to make me groggy and sleepy most of the time and also gave me a cough. These unwelcome effects got worse and worse until I realized I would have to stop using pot. So I made a resolution to quit completely.

Well, it surprised me to find that wasn't so easy. It took me three years of trying before I really gave up smoking marijuana, even though I no longer got pleasant effects from it. I never realized how much of a habit I had and how hooked I was on it. I was certainly abusing the stuff. I think I'd better just stay off it for good now. I'm afraid that if I tried to use it once in a while, my smoking would just creep back up to that addictive level, and I'd be in the same spot as before.

I don't have bad feelings about pot. I learned a lot from it and never really got hurt by it. I think it should be legalized. I also think people who use it should be aware that it can have strong effects and can be addicting if you don't watch out.

— forty-one-year-old man, lawyer

Marijuana and Driving

You want to know about marijuana and driving?

When I first tried driving when stoned, it was pretty weird. I would imagine I was cruising along at fifty miles per hour but would only be going twenty. Sometimes I'd feel as if I were very, very tiny behind a gigantic steering wheel. Going through a long tunnel, I thought I was driving vertically down a shaft into the earth. These illusions were both scary and fun. I never had an accident, but I'm a good driver to begin with and was always careful. I can see where pot could be dangerous for someone not used to it.

One time, while I was in college, I was very stoned late at night in Cleveland and had to drive home. I was going through deserted streets in residential neighborhoods. Suddenly, I couldn't remember whether I was in Cleveland or Pittsburgh, where I grew up. I could turn the scene through the window into either city. Then I came to an intersection that was very familiar, only I had to turn left if it was Cleveland and right if it was Pittsburgh. That's the kind of mind tricks pot can play on you at the wheel.

Later, when I had been smoking marijuana for several years, I never had such strong effects anymore, and driving after smoking was pretty routine for me. A number of times I almost had accidents because joints fell apart on me while I was driving or because lighting a pipe behind the wheel took my attention (and hands) off the wheel. Those hazards were more dangerous than direct effects of the drug.

Finally, pot started making me really sleepy and groggy a lot, and that was a problem for driving, especially when I was by myself on a long haul. I'd think, Boy, it would be nice to smoke a joint, this ride is really boring. So I'd light up and feel pleasantly high for ten minutes or so, then spend the next two hours fighting off the nods. It was no different from getting sleepy normally, but that sure is risky on an interstate highway for you and other people if you don't pull off at a rest stop and either take a nap or somehow wake yourself up.

— thirty-two-year-old man, lab technician

Marijuana as Medicine

Twenty years ago I suddenly developed a paralysis of the right side of my body that baffled the doctors. After ten months it began to improve, but I also lost my vision, and that came back only in part. They finally were able to make a diagnosis of multiple sclerosis.

About three years later I discovered marijuana. A friend told me it was relaxing. My main problem then, aside from partial blindness, was tenseness and tremors in my muscles. Pot cured it, and I've smoked regularly ever since, about four to five times a week. If I go without it for a week, the muscle tremors come back.

Medical science has nothing to offer me. Most people with MS have repeated attacks and keep losing body function. I'm convinced that pot has kept me in remission all these years. It can't help my vision, because there was permanent nerve damage. Still, I can get around fairly well. It does keep my muscles in great shape. I lift weights regularly and feel pretty strong.

I can't believe that marijuana is not legally available for medical use, that a doctor can't prescribe it for me. I want to see it legalized, and I want the government to supply me with it. I'm a veteran and think I ought to get my pot from the VA hospital.

— forty-one-year-old man, part-time roofer

Inhaling Gasoline

One of the best descriptions of gasoline sniffing as it actually occurs was published in 1955 by the late A. E. ("Tajar") Hamilton of the Hamilton School in Sheffield, Mass., in his classic account of children at work and play, *Psychology and the Great God Fun*. One day when the other children had gone on an expedition, Tajar Hamilton reports, he found a boy nicknamed Bullet with a can of gasoline and a gasoline-soaked rag. After a few preliminary questions, Tajar (with Bullet's consent) turned on a recorder and preserved the dialogue for posterity.

TAJAR: Bullet, you said you would come up to the attic and tell me about the gasoline and the bicycles. Will you talk your story into the mike, just as you remember it?

BULLET: Well, I was awful mad when they said I couldn't go on the trip. Sure I picked up the axe when Martha told me not to, but I put it back again. Then she said I couldn't go, and Donnie was going, and when they all went I didn't have anything to do to have fun and I began to get madder and madder all the time. It made me feel kind of sick to be so mad, so I went where they keep the gasoline can and I started to smell it.

TAJAR: What made you want to smell gas, Bullet?

BULLET: Well, when you feel bad, you smell it and it makes you feel kind of hot and kind of drowsy, like you was floating through the air. It makes you feel sort of hot inside and different from the way you were before.

TAJAR: And after you smelled the gas and felt better, what did you do?

BULLET: Then I began to feel mad again and had to do something, so I found a nail. It was an old rusty one, and I got a piece of board to push it with so it wouldn't hurt my hand, and I made holes in all the tires except Donnie's.

TAJAR: Why not in Donnie's?

BULLET: Because they're solid and you can't . . .

TAJAR: And after you had punched all those holes what did you do?

BULLET: Mary hollered to come to dinner, so I went and we had hot dogs at the council ring and then we had some games and then I didn't feel so good, so I went and smelled the gas again.

TAJAR: How long have you liked to smell gas, Bullet?

BULLET: Well, here at camp, ever since about two weeks after I came to the farm. I showed Donnie how to smell it. It makes you feel like you was in fairyland or somewhere else than where you are . . .

TAJAR: Bullet, how come so much gas was spilled on the cellar floor?

BULLET: Oh, I just wanted to get more on my rag. If you have a lot it makes you sort of dream. It gets all dark and you see shooting stars in it, and this time I saw big flies flying in it. They were big and green and had white wings.

TAJAR: And you feel better about yourself and about people after you have one of those dreams?

BULLET: Yep, until I begin to feel bad again, or get mad.

TAJAR: Okay, Bullet, that's all for now. Thank you for being so truthful with me.

> — from *Licit and Illicit Drugs,*
> by Edward M. Brecher
> and the editors of *Consumer Reports* (1972)

Poppers in the Pool

I was first introduced to amyl nitrite during my senior year in college. The father of one of my friends had a heart condition for which he used the drug. He would amass huge numbers of poppers and give them out to anyone who wanted them. I had read of this drug but had no firsthand experience with it.

My friends and I used to get together on weekends and hang out in a heated pool with a whirlpool bath in the condominium complex where I lived. One cool December evening after drinking several glasses of wine, we got into the near-scalding, frothing waters of the pool. I was already warm from the alcohol and wondered what it would be like to dilate my arteries all the way. I suggested we try a popper. I broke one and inhaled deeply, filling my lungs with the stong odor.

The effect was immediate. My arms and legs felt like liquid warmth, and at the same time I got a pounding in my head. (We came to call this the "jackhammer effect.") When I exhaled, my vision blurred, with small blue patches filling my field of vision. I then jumped in the nearby unheated swimming pool and got an even brighter visual display. All the effects lasted only a few minutes. I liked them enough to repeat this ritual many times in the course of the evening. In fact, I did it over and over on many evenings.

I never knew about sexual uses of poppers until much later, when a gay friend told me about it. I never got into that. My interest was just in the spectacular rush and sensory fireworks. After a few months of doing poppers in the whirlpool bath, I guess I lost interest in having the same experience over and over. Maybe I just overdid it to the point where it started to get boring. In any case, all that was three years ago, and I haven't used amyl nitrite since.

— twenty-year-old man, medical student

In Datura Country

I was on a camping trip with a friend in northern Arizona in remote canyon country. We noticed a lot of datura plants growing around us, some with seed pods. When we ran out of marijuana, I suggested that we try datura. Neither Tom nor I had ever done it.

We each ate about ten seeds and drank a cup of tea made from the leaves. That was just after sunset. We started a small campfire, although it was a warm night, and sat around waiting for something to happen. After about an hour we both started to feel different. I got restless and walked away from the fire into some big boulders at the base of a cliff.

You have to understand that what I'm going to tell you from this point on is not a clear memory. It's more like trying to put together the pieces of a dream. I have some very vivid pictures in my mind, but they don't all hang together in a logical order, and there are definite holes in my memory.

Anyway, I think I found a comfortable place in the rocks and sort of curled up with my eyes closed. Then I remember seeing bats, a lot of bats and very large ones. They kept flying at me, coming right in close. Their faces were hideous. I thought to myself, "I've never seen bats like that." I wanted to find Tom to see what he made of them, but when I got up I couldn't tell where I was. It didn't look like Arizona anymore, and Tom was nowhere in sight.

I was in a dark forest, or maybe a swamp. It was hot, and the air was thick and hard to breathe. I couldn't tell if it was day or night. I kept getting tangled in these vines and roots and had to fight my way through them to make any progress. Also, there were dark shapes moving in and out of the trees that seemed to follow me, but I couldn't get a good look at them to see what they were. They did not seem friendly. I remember feeling very thirsty, trying to find water, getting more hung up in the undergrowth.

I came to some sort of pool. The water was black and stagnant, and I wasn't sure I should drink it. I scooped some up and put it to my lips. It was warm and thick, not at all refreshing. Then I realized it was blood. That made me think I was going to die. I fell on the ground and started crying. The black shapes got nearer and bigger. I still couldn't see what they were, but I knew they were waiting for me to die so they could devour me. It seemed like an eternity as they closed in.

The next thing I remember is waking up in a burning desert, nothing but sand. I was tied to a stake, left to die of thirst. The sun beat down on me unbearably. I tried to call for help but couldn't make any sound. That also seemed to go on forever.

Then I discovered I was in the rocks just a short distance from our campsite. The sun was up; it must have been ten o'clock. My mouth and throat were completely parched. The light hurt my eyes, and I couldn't focus them. I felt very hung over. Then I remembered eating the datura and was able to sort out some of the weird dreams or whatever they were.

Tom was nowhere in sight. I tried shouting for him but my throat was so dry I couldn't yell very loud, and drinking water didn't help much. I searched the immediate area and eventually found Tom stumbling around. He had no clothes on and was pretty cut up. He didn't know where he was and couldn't tell me what had happened. I got him cleaned up and made sure he didn't have any serious injuries. He slept off and on for the next few hours, then came to himself, although he was hung over even worse than I was. He had no memory of anything after eating the datura. All he could say was that he thought he'd stick to marijuana from now on.

— twenty-three-year-old man, ranch hand

I Ate the Panther Amanita

On two occasions I ate the panther mushroom. I was living out in the woods in western Oregon. I once ate *Amanita muscaria*, but did not get much effect from it, just a little sick feeling. Word went around that the panther would make you high. Most of my friends were afraid to try the panther. I decided to be the guinea pig. I found a medium-sized specimen, sliced it, and steeped it in hot water and lemon juice. Then I drank the liquid and ate half the mushroom.

About forty minutes later I was feeling dreamy and relaxed. I lay on my back in the woods and saw images with my eyes closed. There was no sickness and generally no bad effects. The dreamy state lasted about three hours.

That experience encouraged me to experiment further, so a week later I ate twice as much, prepared in the same way. The dreamy state came on faster and was more intense. After an hour I tried to get up but felt very confused and disoriented. I didn't know whether I was dreaming or awake or what was real. It wasn't scary, just strange.

I crawled out on a big fallen tree over a pond, and while trying to find a good position, fell off. Then I wasn't sure if it had happened or not, so I got back up on the tree and fell off again. I kept having a compulsion to repeat the fall, because I couldn't tell if it had happened or was going to happen. On about the seventh time, I hit my head on some rocks and was bleeding pretty badly. Some people saw me and got scared. I guess I looked bad, although I was unaware of being hurt. They drove me an hour to the nearest emergency hospital. By the time I got there I thought I had died and gone to heaven. I thought the doctors and nurses were angels and started singing hymns. They did not know what to make of me.

They kept me for a while and made sure I hadn't fractured my skull, then let me go, all patched up. I was coming back to normal when they sent me away, about eight hours after eating the mushroom. My face got all black and blue from the fall, but otherwise I was all right.

I haven't eaten panther *Amanitas* since then. I'm still interested to try again, but I would want to have someone with me to watch out for me, and I think I would take less than that last time.

— thirty-one-year-old man, unemployed

Positive Experiences with PCP

I've had very positive experiences with PCP, which, I guess, makes me unusual, since everyone says it's a terrible drug. I used it over a few months about five years ago. It used to come sprayed on dried parsley leaves that were then rolled into very thin joints. From one to three tokes on one of these joints would give me a high lasting four to ten hours. My consciousness would alter within a minute of taking the first toke.

PCP would make me very flexible, allowing me to be active or restful. I could jog farther and longer than normal under its influence or I could sit still and meditate. I could close my eyes and create inner visions, sometimes seeing colorful, changing, geometric designs, as if I had ingested mushrooms or peyote.

For years I have suffered lower back pains, supposedly due to the deterioration of cartilage between my lumbar and sacral vertebrae. Whenever I smoked PCP I felt no pain, and as I've said, could jog comfortably. Even after the drug wore off, I experienced no pain from any athletic activities I performed. A few times I jogged in six-inch snow wearing only sneakers and shorts without getting cold. Even when I got back to the house after such a run, my friends noted that my skin was not at all cold.

My thinking was often imaginative and lucid. And I laughed a lot. I would often laugh so much that people around me, even though they didn't know what I was laughing at (I don't remember now, myself) would also start laughing. I remember doubling over and sometimes rolling on the floor in fits of laughter. I loved every second of it.

Finally, there was a strange "psychic" effect of PCP, which I still don't understand. Once in a while under the influence of the drug, I would feel as though a "ray" or "beam" entered my head through the back; I can't really describe it. When this happened, I would have thoughts or knowledge that I would later find were telepathic or pre-cognitive. I would receive a thought from a friend or realize something would happen in the future. One night I described to a friend a drug bust that we would be involved in and the aftermath of it in months to follow. It all happened exactly as I predicted.

Maybe these experiences were just cases of heightened intuitive power. My unconscious mind might have had all the information to make these predictions, but it took the drug, or the altered state brought about by the drug, to put the information together and let it come to the surface. I don't know, but that "ray" or "beam" feeling always came first, and when it occurred, I would say to myself or to a friend, kind of nodding my head and rolling my eyes somewhat in jest, "Here we go again." I wondered if I were a psychonaut or just a plain psychic nut. Whatever, it was fun.

My use of angel dust, as I called it, finally got out of hand. I was taking it all the time, and people around me told me I was acting too crazily. So I stopped and haven't used it since. Sometime, I'd like to experiment with it again to explore those physical and mental powers it seems to release in me.

— thirty-six-year-old man, screenwriter

Nothing Good About PCP

I've tried most drugs and think most have their place. PCP is one of the few I can see nothing good about. I've taken it in pill form a few times, thinking it was pure THC. One time I was about to give a lecture to a large group of medical doctors. I was using marijuana a lot then and went outside just before the talk to smoke a joint. Someone I didn't know came along and produced a joint. He lit it and handed it to me. I took a deep drag on it and only noticed the taste of PCP after I had the smoke in my lungs. I couldn't believe that anyone would do that to me, but before I could say anything, I was called in to the auditorium to start my lecture.

On the way to the podium, I started rushing on the PCP. I could hardly control my legs or thoughts, and could only get words out of my mouth with great difficulty. If I hadn't been experienced with drugs, I would really have lost it. As it was, I don't think anyone really noticed. It probably seemed that I was just talking pretty slowly for the first five minutes; after that I got myself together and was able to control the drug. I was furious, however, and when I finished, I found the guy that slipped me that loaded joint and told him what I thought of him. I've never seen him since, and I've never taken any PCP since, either.

— thirty-seven-year-old man, medical doctor

Ketamine Summer

Soon after I began work in a pharmacology lab, I met a coworker who shared my desire to alter ordinary consciousness by means of drugs. One summer day during our lunch break, he handed me the package insert from a box of ketamine. After reading the precautions warning of possible hallucinations, delirium, and dissociative states, we decided to try it that evening.

We wanted to inject a subanesthetic dose, but neither of us knew how to calculate a "recreational" dose or how to give injections. In retrospect, I believe it was this uncertainty that made our first trip on ketamine one of the best. Robert shot first, injecting the drug into the muscle of his leg. Then I took about twice as much, injecting it into my arm muscle.

Within five minutes of the injection I came on to the drug. At first, all my organs felt like lead, especially my stomach, and I thought I might have to vomit. These physical sensations quickly gave way to an incredible dreamlike state. I lay down and tried to talk, but my words were garbled, and my mouth felt numb. There also seemed to be a delay between speaking and hearing what I said, so that I kept repeating myself in a vain attempt to "catch up" and hear what I just said.

The brick walls of the room began to vibrate. I had to close my eyes to avoid another round of nausea. With my eyes closed I entered a new dimension, filled with multicolored triangles, rotating clockwise. When I tried to get up and walk, the floor heaved up and down, reminiscent of a boat on a stormy sea. I sat down and felt detached from my physical being, lapsing into a state of semiconsciousness. This lasted for what seemed like hours, but by the time I returned to near-normal reality, only forty-five minutes had passed since the injection.

This first experience inspired Robert and me to repeat our explorations with ketamine. We took it every day for the next two months. It was an interesting time. I haven't used the drug since then.

— twenty-five-year-old man, laboratory technician

Addicted to Cough Pills

I've had asthma all my life and am allergic to just about everything. Allergic skin rashes and asthma are my biggest problems. I've been in the hospital for the asthma a lot of times and to control it I have to take a lot of medication, including cortisone and pills for coughing.

As a child I took a lot of codeine for coughs. For the past ten years I've been on Hycodan, which I understand contains a narcotic [hydrocodone]. Originally, I took one tablet four times a day; now I take two four times a day. If I try to cut down the dose I start coughing and get really congested. Also, I get upset and can't sleep.

If I think about it, I guess I know I'm addicted, but I don't like to face that. I've never had anything to do with drugs, and no one in my family or people I work with would think of me as an addict. Most doctors give me the Hycodan without asking too many questions, but sometimes I've gone to several different ones to get enough prescriptions so that I wouldn't have to worry about running out. I know I should try to stop the Hycodan, but I don't think I can face the day without it. I don't know what I can do.

— fifty-two-year-old woman, university guidance counselor

The Wonders of Sudafed

I suspect most people take antihistamines just because they have been brainwashed by the pharmaceutical industry. I concluded long ago that I would much rather put up with the symptoms of a cold than endure the depression antihistamines give me.

Two summers ago, I came down with a head cold just as a low pressure system settled over the East Coast. The combination caused one of my ears to close up. After a day or so of constant tugging at my ear, it was becoming sore. I consulted my local pharmacist, who, hearing of my aversion to antihistamines, recommended Sudafed. I had never heard of it.

The Sudafed worked wonders right away, drying up my sinuses and unblocking the congested ear without producing any of the hated side effects of antihistamines. It also really zapped me — better than coffee. In fact, Sudafed is so stimulating that, though I now use it whenever I have a cold, I can't take it too late in the day, or I won't be able to fall asleep that night. I think it's a great drug and am surprised more people don't know about it.

— forty-year-old housewife

Cotton Poisoning

Cotton poisoning is the term used to describe the body's reaction to a particle of fiber, like cotton, or of some other foreign substance that gets injected into the bloodstream. It usually appears in two to four hours after injection and causes muscle cramps, chills, cold sweats, and nausea. After two or three hours of discomfort, it usually passes away, leaving the victim exhausted.

This is my understanding of cotton poisoning after talking to people who have experienced it and after experiencing it myself. My own reaction was different in that it kept recurring. I still don't understand it.

One night I was with two friends, and we were shooting some drug. I don't remember whether it was Demerol, Dilaudid, or heroin that we were using, but it was something of that nature. We put the drug in a spoon and used steaming hot water to dilute it; then we drew the liquid into a syringe through a piece of cigarette filter. We all used the same needle, and we cleaned it thoroughly between uses with steaming hot water. Everything was done in the normal fashion and we all got high.

After about two and a half hours I began to feel cold. I turned off the cooler and put on an extra shirt, and I felt a little better. It didn't take long before I was cold again. I asked my friends if they, too, were cold, but they said they were very warm.

I got colder and colder and broke out in goose bumps. I began to shiver and break out in a sweat. My muscles were very tense from the coldness, and I felt as if I was waiting for a bus in a windy snowstorm without a coat. I was clutching at my chest, shivering, and the muscles in my back and shoulders began to cramp from being so tense. Then I started to sweat very heavily and began vomiting. My head was spinning and throbbing. I didn't know what was going on.

One of my friends said I had cotton poisoning. He said that he had had it before and there was no way of stopping it. It would probably last another hour or two. He went into the bathroom and ran a hot bath for me — that was the only thing that would help, he said. It did help some. I was still cold, but the hot water relieved the backache. I kept sweating and throwing up, though. I don't know how long it took, but I was finally able to get out of the tub and go to bed, completely exhausted.

The next day I was okay, but the day after the whole thing came back, just the same, and I hadn't shot any more drugs, just smoked a lot of pot and drank beer. Over the next few days, I kept having recurrences and they kept getting worse. I thought I was going to die a few times. No one had ever heard of cotton poisoning recurring like that. I finally went to a doctor, but he had never even heard of cotton poisoning, and I had to explain it to him. He was no help at all. Finally, after I got sick every other day for a week, the whole thing went away. I've never had it since.

I've had some bad experiences with drugs. I've had some really bad times with opium in India, including miserable highs and terrible chest pains. I've done hallucinogens that were so strange I once lay down in a bonfire. I've been so wiped out on the combination of morphine and amphetamines that I've lost track of days at a time and regained consciousness in awful situations. Except for my being sent to prison, no drug experience or drug-related experience has been so hard to deal with, so unpleasant, and so painful as my episode of cotton poisoning.

— twenty-three-year-old man, prisoner

Panic Reactions

As a doctor interested in drug reactions, I've had occasion to treat many cases of drug panic. I worked in an emergency room in San Francisco during the big, early days of pot and acid, and used to see all kinds of people come in thinking they were going crazy or dying. I soon learned that these reactions were more psychological than pharmacological.

One time, a father and mother came in with their teen-age daughter. The girl was a pot smoker and had been pressuring her mother to try it. Finally, the mother agreed, but, since she didn't know how to smoke, the daughter baked up some pot brownies. The mother ate one. An hour later she was hysterical, thinking she had been poisoned and was losing her mind. Meanwhile, the daughter had eaten three brownies and just felt very high. Before I had a chance to do anything, a staff psychiatrist came down and got caught up in the family hysteria. (The father, who had come home from work early, was the worst of the three, pleading with us to save his wife.) The psychiatrist gave the mother an injection of Thorazine and admitted her to the psychiatric ward. She stayed agitated and panicked for four days. I could have talked her down in an hour, if I had just been able to get her away from her husband and calm her.

The best method I hit upon for dealing with drug panics in the emergency room was to let the patients know I did not consider their problems serious. When a couple of teen-agers would come in with a stricken friend, I'd just say, "Okay, have a seat and relax. I'll be with you as soon as I can." Then I'd mostly ignore them. When they demanded attention for the crisis, I'd say, "Look, there are people here who really have things wrong with them that I have to deal with. Your friend is just upset and all he needs is to calm down. So get him to breathe deeply and regularly, and I'll come back as soon as I take care of the real problems in here."

Usually, by the time I'd come back, the victim would be looking better, and the whole group would just want to make a graceful exit from the hospital. Of course, if it's an older person thinking they are dying of a heart attack or something, you should go through the motions of examining them and telling them firmly that their physical health is fine. I never give tranquilizers or sedatives to panic victims, just reassurance and calming vibes. The worst thing you can do is give the impression that you think something is really wrong.

— forty-year-old man, general practitioner

Different Tastes in Drugs

My husband and I met in college in the late 1960s. We were both involved in antiwar politics and did some experimenting with group living and using drugs, mostly marijuana and psychedelics. I found the experiences interesting, but after a while did not want to repeat them frequently. My husband, on the other hand, thought marijuana was the greatest thing he had ever discovered. Smoking it became an important ritual for him.

Over the years he's continued to smoke it. Once in a while, I join him, but I've come to find I don't like the effect all that much. I can't concentrate well when I'm stoned and sometimes feel mentally scattered and vulnerable. I guess my drug of choice is wine. Two glasses of good wine put me in just the right state after a trying day. John drinks wine, too, but for getting high he prefers marijuana.

In the past few years, our different preferences in drugs have become a problem for us. My not liking marijuana separates me from John's closest friends and weakens our relationship. I don't think married people have to do everything together, but this is something important, and my inability to share John's highs bothers me. Also, I find I resent his smoking friends, since I'm the outsider, the "straight wife," when they are around. Yet I know that if I object, I will just drive him out of the house to get high with them elsewhere.

We try to talk about our problem but have not come up with an answer. I just don't like marijuana and he does. It may seem like a little matter, but when we are having a hard time with each other, it comes to symbolize all of the differences that keep us from sharing fully with each other, and I can see it harming our marriage. I don't know other couples who have this problem.

— thirty-five-year-old housewife

A Mother's Concern

Even though my son has a learning disability, which always made things hard for him at school, it never occurred to me while he was growing up that he wouldn't turn out all right in the end. Now, however, I'm not so sure. In the three years since he first became involved with drugs, starting at age fourteen, he has been arrested twice (for bizarre behavior) and hospitalized three times, the last time for a period of more than eight months. Although his severe problems began when he first tried LSD, now even pot can trigger a psychotic episode.

Unlike his friends, and even his younger brother, my son cannot handle drugs. For him they are simply poisons. He knows this. And yet the social pressure on him to take drugs is often more than he can withstand. Despite his history and my repeated appeals, his friends continue to supply him with drugs, even going so far as to smuggle them into the hospital the last time he was there.

— forty-five-year-old housewife

The Ecstasy of Love

Where, like a pillow on a bed,
  A Pregnant banke swel'd up, to rest
The violet's reclining head,
  Sat we two, one anothers best.
Our hands were firmely cimented
  With a fast balme, which thence did spring,
Our eye-beames twisted, and did thred
  Our eyes, upon one double string;
So to'entergraft our hands, as yet
  Was all the meanes to make us one,
And pictures in our eyes to get
  Was all our propagation.
As 'twixt two equal Armies, Fate
  Suspends uncertaine victorie,
Our soules, (which to advance their state,
  Were gone out,) hung 'twixt her, and mee.
And whil'st our soules negotiate there,
  Wee like sepulchrall statues lay;
All day, the same our postures were,
  And wee said nothing all the day.

— from "The Extasie" by John Donne (1572–1631)

Speaking in Tongues

I speak in tongues. This other language gives me the words my spirit needs to express itself. It happens on two different kinds of occasions. One occurs when I am depressed, anxious, upset, or feel a great sorrow in my heart and don't really know exactly what is wrong. Speaking releases all that bottled-up tension and depression. I also find myself wanting to speak in tongues when I feel really good. I want to express the tremendous love or peace or wonder I feel but can't find words for.

When I speak in tongues it is as if a voice from within me is talking. Another part of my being — beyond conscious thought — takes over and lets me express what my inner spirit is feeling in a language all its own. I am totally in the here and now when this happens, not worrying about the past or dreaming about the future. The feeling is similar to what some people get from psychedelic drugs. No other reality exists beyond what I am a part of at that moment.

I received "the gift of tongues" (as the Bible calls it) while I was involved with a Christian commune. This group believes tongues is a gift from the Holy Spirit to permit fellowship with the Father. It means believers have direct access to God.

I was once in a remote wilderness area of British Columbia on a canoe trip. In a marshy area around a lake our group came across big tracks, perhaps of moose or elk. I suddenly felt thrilled to be among wild animals, where man had not destroyed nature. I looked up to see mountains and sky stretch to infinity. I suddenly realized how beautiful the world I live in can be. Then I started to speak in tongues. As I did, I lost my sense of self-consciousness and with it my feelings of loneliness, isolation, and alienation from the rest of the world. I felt connected to all of life.

Speaking in tongues makes me high. It makes me experience an altered state of consciousness. It lets me glimpse another reality — infinite realities — beyond the scope of my "normal" state of consciousness.

Speaking in tongues resembles meditation. One has to come to it with the proper set and setting, to be in tune. I am sure many Christians who speak in tongues feel the release of an emotional burden or, as in Pentecostal churches, a real high; but to have the total here and now experience, one has to come with a desire for it. Tongues is not magic in itself. The magic is in using tongues to open oneself to powers already within each of us.

— thirty-year-old housewife

Cross-referenced entries are in *italics*.

Abscess A localized collection of pus surrounded by an inflamed area, often the result of a bacterial infection.

Abstinence Refraining from using something, such as a drug, by one's own choice. In pharmacology the term "abstinence syndrome" is equivalent to *withdrawal* syndrome.

Abusers People who use drugs in ways that threaten their health or impair their social or economic functioning.

Acetic acid The acid in vinegar.

Acid Slang term for LSD (lysergic acid diethylamide).

Active principle The main chemical constituent of a drug plant. Cocaine, for example, is the active principle of coca leaf. Although active principles may be responsible for many of the effects of drug plants, they do not exactly reproduce those effects and in pure form have higher toxicity and potential for abuse.

Acupuncture An ancient Chinese system of medical treatment that aims to influence energy flow around the body by inserting needles into particular points on the skin.

Acute Intense and of short duration, as opposed to *chronic*.

Addiction In reference to drugs, a pattern of consumption marked by compulsive taking of a drug, the need for increasing doses over time to maintain the same effect (*tolerance*), and the appearance of symptoms when the drug is stopped that disappear when it is reinstated (*withdrawal*).

Adulteration The deliberate addition of impurities to a pure substance — for example, the cutting of cocaine with sugars and cheap *local anesthetics* to make it go further on the black market.

Alkali Any substance that in solution gives a pH of greater than 7.0. Lye (potassium hydroxide or sodium hydroxide), baking soda (sodium bicarbonate), and lime (calcium oxide or calcium hydroxide) are examples of alkalis.

Amnesia   Loss of memory, either partial or total.

Amys   Slang term for amyl nitrite.

Analgesic   A medication that reduces or eliminates pain.

Anemia   A deficiency of red blood cells or hemoglobin, reducing the blood's capacity to carry oxygen.

Angel dust   Slang term for PCP (phencyclidine).

Animal tranquilizer   Slang term for PCP (phencyclidine), because of its use as a veterinary anesthetic.

Antidepressants   Pharmaceutical drugs prescribed for the treatment of persistent and severe *depression*. Imipramine (Tofranil) and amitriptyline (Elavil) are examples.

Antihistamines   A large class of *synthetic drugs* used to relieve allergic symptoms.

Apathy   Lack of feeling, emotion, or interest in what excites most people.

Asphyxiation   Unconsciousness or death resulting from lack of oxygen.

Asthma   A respiratory disease caused by constriction of the bronchial tubes with resultant difficulty in breathing. Wheezing on exhalation is the most characteristic symptom.

Bad trip   An unpleasant experience on a *psychoactive drug*, especially a *hallucinogen*. *Paranoia*, panic, scary *hallucinations*, and *depression* may all occur in a bad trip.

Barbs   Barbiturates, such as secobarbital (Seconal).

Biorhythms   Cyclic changes in biological functions, such as twenty-four-hour cycles of waking and sleeping and secretion of certain hormones, and the monthly menstrual cycle in women.

Bronchitis   *Inflammation* of the bronchial tubes, producing a painful cough and other breathing difficulties.

Bummer   Slang term for an unpleasant experience on a *psychoactive drug*. Similar to *bad trip*.

Burn-out   A condition of emotional and intellectual impairment supposed to be the result of excessive use of *psychoactive drugs*. Also, a person with this condition.

Bust   An arrest, especially for involvement with illegal drugs. Also used as a verb.

Cellulose   An indigestible carbohydrate that is the main structural component of all plant tissues and fibers.

Chamomile   A low-growing plant of the daisy family with yellow flowers and a pleasant applelike smell. The dried flowers make a relaxing tea that also alleviates indigestion.

Chemotherapy   The treatment of cancer by giving patients very toxic drugs that kill growing cells, in the hope that more cancerous cells will die than normal ones.

Chipping The practice of using *narcotics* such as heroin on an occasional basis without developing true *addiction*.

Chronic Persisting over time, as opposed to *acute*.

Coke Slang term for cocaine. (Others are "blow" and "snow.")

Coma Deep and prolonged unconsciousness, usually the result of disease, injury, or poisoning.

Controlled substances Plants and chemicals listed in the Federal Controlled Substances Act, the law regulating disapproved psychoactive drugs and those approved only for medical use.

Convulsion An intense episode of muscle contraction, usually caused by abnormal brain function.

Cop To obtain a supply of a desired drug. Same as *score*.

Cornea The transparent, outer covering of the eye, overlying the iris, pupil, and lens.

Crash To experience *depression*, *lethargy*, or sleepiness after a drug-induced *high*, especially common after using *stimulants*.

Cut To *adulterate* a drug by adding to it some substance to make it go further. Also, any substance used for this purpose.

Deal To sell or distribute illegal drugs.

Deliriants Drugs that cause *delirium*. Datura is an example.

Delirium A state of mental confusion marked by disorientation and *hallucinations*. Fever and certain drugs are common causes.

Depressants Drugs that reduce the activity of the nervous system. Alcohol, *downers*, and *narcotics* are all depressants.

Depression Melancholy mood; dejection.

Detoxify To recover from the action of a toxin on the system. For example, treatment programs exist to help addicts detoxify from opiates — that is, to stop taking the drugs and adjust to being non-users.

Dope 1) Psychoactive drugs in general, especially illegal ones. 2) Specific drugs or types of drugs, usually opiates, *downers*, or marijuana.

Down 1) No longer under the effect of a *psychoactive drug*, especially a *stimulant* or *hallucinogen*, as in, "If you take *acid* now, you won't be down till after midnight." 2) Depressed, as in, "I'm feeling really down."

Downers Barbiturates, minor tranquilizers, and related *depressants*.

D.T.'s Delirium tremens — the most severe form of *withdrawal* from alcohol, marked by agitation, *hallucinations*, and other mental and physical imbalances.

Duster A PCP-laced *joint* (from *angel dust*, a slang term for PCP).

Ejaculation In males, the discharge of seminal fluid, usually during orgasm.

Emaciated Thin and gaunt, as from starvation or illness.

Emphysema A *chronic* respiratory disease in which lung tissue loses its elasticity and with it the ability to exchange carbon dioxide for oxygen. Patients with emphysema suffer from progressively diminishing breathing capacity and may eventually become bedridden "respiratory cripples."

Endogenous drugs   Drugs produced within the body.

Enzyme   A protein produced by a living organism that catalyzes (speeds up) biochemical reactions. Many digestive enzymes enable the body to process foods, for example.

Estrogen   One of a group of hormones, mostly manufactured by the ovaries in women, responsible for producing female sex characteristics and regulating fertility.

Euphoria   A feeling of great happiness or well-being.

Fix   Slang term for a dose of a mood-altering drug, especially an intravenous dose of an opiate, as in, "I need a fix." Also used as a verb, as in, "When did you fix last?"

Flashback   A recurrence of symptoms associated with LSD or other *hallucinogens* some time after the actual drug experience.

Freak out   To panic or lose emotional control.

Freebase   A smokable form of cocaine. As a verb, to smoke cocaine in this form.

GABA   Gamma-amino-butyric acid, a simple, organic chemical that serves as a neurotransmitter in certain brain cells. Its effect is inhibitory and depressing of nervous function.

Gas   Slang term for nitrous oxide.

Gastrointestinal tract   The whole chain of tubular structures from the mouth to the anus concerned with the processing of food.

Gram   A unit of mass and weight in the metric system, defined as one thousandth of a kilogram. (A kilogram is about 2.2 pounds.)

Hallucination   The perception of something that is not there, such as seeing pink elephants or hearing voices that other people cannot hear; also the nonperception of objects or events that are perceived by others (negative hallucination). Hallucinations can be symptoms of physical or mental illness, or the result of taking some kinds of *psychoactive* drugs.

Hallucinogens   Drugs that stimulate the nervous system and produce varied changes in perception and mood. Examples are LSD, DMT, mescaline, and *magic mushrooms*. Hallucinogens are also known as psychedelics.

Hash   Slang term for hashish, the concentrated resin of the marijuana plant.

Hash oil   A dark, syrupy liquid obtained by extracting the resin of marijuana with solvents and concentrating it.

Head   A person who uses *psychoactive drugs*, especially marijuana (a *pot* head) or *psychedelics* (such as an *acid* head).

Head shops   Stores that sell drug-related products, such as smoking devices, drug literature, and other materials.

Hepatitis *Inflammation* of the liver, usually because of infection with a virus. Jaundice, weakness, and digestive problems are common symptoms that may last for weeks or months. There is no specific treatment.

High An altered state of consciousness, marked by *euphoria*, feelings of lightness, self-transcendence, and energy. High states are not necessarily drug-related. They may occur spontaneously or in response to various activities that affect mood, perception, and concentration. Also used as an adjective.

Hog Slang term for PCP (phencyclidine).

Hormone A chemical substance produced by one organ of the body, such as a gland, and conveyed, usually by the blood, to another organ (or organs), where it exerts a controlling or regulating action. Insulin is a hormone produced by the pancreas that regulates sugar metabolism throughout the body.

Hyperventilation Abnormally rapid, deep breathing.

Hypothermia The condition of abnormally low body temperature, usually the result of exposure to cold. Early symptoms are uncontrollable shivering and bizarre changes in consciousness. If not treated, it can progress to coma and death.

Immune system Those organs and tissues of the body concerned with the recognition and destruction of foreign substances, such as invading germs. The immune system includes organs such as the spleen and tonsils along with the bone marrow and certain white blood cells.

Inflammation A characteristic response of the body to irritation, injury, and infection. It consists of swelling, warmth, redness, and pain in the affected part.

Insomnia Inability to sleep.

Intoxication The state of being under the influence of a poison or drug, with effects ranging from stimulation and exhilaration to stupefaction and loss of consciousness.

Intramuscular Within a muscle, such as the injection of a drug into the muscle of an arm or leg.

Intravenous Within a vein, such as the injection of a drug directly into the bloodstream.

Joint A marijuana cigarette.

Junk Slang term for *narcotics*, especially heroin.

Junkie A heroin addict.

Laughing gas Slang term for nitrous oxide.

Lethargy A state of sluggish indifference or unhealthy drowsiness.

Leukemia A form of cancer marked by uncontrolled multiplication of white blood cells.

Local anesthetic A substance that blocks transmission of pain by nerves when injected into a part of the body or when applied to mucous membranes. Procaine is a synthetic local anesthetic marketed under the brand name Novocain.

Look-alike drugs   Tablets and capsules made to resemble pharmaceutical *stimulants* and *depressants,* such as amphetamines and Quaalude; sold on the black market or in *head shops.*

Ludes   Tablets of methaqualone (Quaalude).

Magic mushrooms   Mushrooms that contain the natural *hallucinogen* psilocybin.

Mainline   To inject a drug *intravenously.*

Menopause   In females, the permanent cessation of the menstrual cycle, usually occurring around age fifty.

Messed up   Strongly intoxicated on a drug.

Metabolism   All the physical and chemical processes involved in the maintenance of life.

Microgram   One millionth of a *gram.*

Milligram   One thousandth of a *gram.*

Mood drugs   *Psychoactive drugs* in general, especially *stimulants* and *depressants.*

Multiple sclerosis   An incurable disease of the central nervous system marked by progressive degeneration of the insulating sheaths of nerve cells and consequent losses of body functions. The cause is unknown.

Mystic   One who aims for union with the divine by means of deep meditation. Mystics believe in realities other than the one perceived by the ordinary senses.

Narcotics   A class of *depressant* drugs derived from opium or related chemically to compounds in opium. Regular use of narcotics often leads to *addiction.*

Neurochemical   A chemical substance produced by nerves and involved in the transmission of information by nerves.

OD   Overdose, used as both a noun and a verb, as in, "Anyone who *shoots* drugs should know how to avoid an OD," and, "The last time I took a *downer* I OD'd on it."

OTC   Over-the-counter, referring to drugs sold legally without prescription.

Paranoia   Delusions of persecution or grandeur; unreasoning belief that one is the target of conspiracies and patterns of events aimed at one's destruction or benefit. In common usage, the term is a synonym for extreme fear, especially of other people and situations.

Paraquat   A chemical herbicide used to kill unwanted plants. In recent years government agencies have sprayed it from the air on marijuana fields, especially in Mexico.

Pineal gland   A tiny, light-sensitive organ in the center of the brain, also called the pineal eye or "third eye." In reptiles it controls changes in skin color. In humans it is a master gland of the endocrine system, probably regulating many *biorhythms*.

Polydrug use   The consumption of more than one drug at the same time.

Pop   To swallow a drug in pill form.

Poppers   Slang term for amyl nitrite.

Pot   Slang term for marijuana. (Others are "grass," "reefer," and "weed.")

Potency   In pharmacology, the measure of relative strength of similar drugs. If a lower dose of drug A produces the same effect as a higher dose of drug B, A is said to be more potent than B.

Prostration   Total exhaustion.

Psychedelics   Synonym for *hallucinogens*.

Psychoactive drugs   Drugs that affect the mind, especially mood, thought, or perception.

Psychosis   Loss of ability to distinguish reality as perceived by others from one's own private mental productions. The most serious category of mental illness, it is often marked by *hallucinations*, delusions, and disturbances of mood.

Reaction time   In psychology, the time interval between the application of a stimulus and the detection of a response. In a simple reaction time test, a subject is asked to press a button as soon as a light flashes.

Recreational drugs   Any drugs used nonmedically for enjoyment or entertainment.

Reflex   A simple nervous circuit. For example, a tendon reflex is initiated by striking a tendon; this stimulus travels to the spinal cord along a single nerve and quickly produces a response in another nerve that causes a contraction in the muscle.

Resin   A sticky substance of plant origin that is insoluble in water.

Respiratory tract   The breathing apparatus of the body, including the nose, throat, bronchial tubes, lungs, and associated structures.

Rheumatism   *Chronic* aches and pains in muscles, joints, and bones, leading to discomfort and disability.

Rip off   To rob, cheat, or take advantage of, such as in a transaction involving drugs. The noun "rip-off" refers to both the actions themselves and the person who does them.

Rush   A sudden, dramatic change in consciousness and body sensation resulting from taking certain *psychoactive drugs* by inhalation or injection.

Schizophrenia   The commonest form of *psychosis*, chiefly affecting thought. It is of unknown cause and is generally considered incurable. Major tranquilizers are the treatment of choice and may allow some schizophrenics to function better.

Score   To obtain a supply of a desired drug. Same as *cop*.

Sedative-hypnotics   A class of *depressants* that induces restfulness in low doses and sleep in higher doses. Alcohol, barbiturates, and the minor tranquilizers make up this class of drugs.

Semisynthetic drugs   Drugs created by chemists from materials found in nature.

Sensory isolation tank   An oblong, lightproof, soundproof tank partially filled with a strong salt solution maintained at body temperature. A person floating in the tank experiences little outside stimulation and can explore inner states. Used for relaxation and meditation as well as to investigate altered states of consciousness.

Set   Expectation, especially unconscious expectation, as a variable determining people's reactions to drugs.

Setting   Environment — physical, social, and cultural — as a variable determining people's reactions to drugs.

Shoot   To inject a drug *intravenously*.

Sinsemilla   High-grade, seedless, flowering tops of marijuana.

Skin-popping   The practice of injecting drugs, especially heroin, *subcutaneously* rather than into a muscle or vein.

Sleeping pills   Barbiturates and related *sedative-hypnotics*.

Sniff   To inhale the fumes of organic solvents to produce changes in consciousness.

Snort   To inhale a powdered drug.

Snuff   1) Finely powdered tobacco, which may be inhaled or placed in the mouth. 2) Any finely powdered drug intended for nasal inhalation. 3) To take a drug in powdered form by nasal inhalation.

Spacy   Detached or disconnected from ordinary reality as a result of using *psychoactive drugs*. (A related term is "spaced out.")

Speed   *Stimulants*, especially amphetamines. (Other slang terms for amphetamines are "crank," "zip," and "crystal.")

Speedball   A combination of a *stimulant* and a *depressant*, especially cocaine and heroin, intended for *intravenous* use.

Spore   A microscopic reproductive cell of lower plants and mushrooms.

Steroids   A large family of pharmaceutical drugs related to the adrenal hormone cortisone.

Stimulants   Drugs that increase the activity of the nervous system, causing wakefulness. Caffeine, cocaine, and amphetamines are examples.

Stoned   1) Intoxicated on a *psychoactive drug*, especially marijuana, 2) Having the nature of consciousness influenced by marijuana and other drugs, as in "stoned humor."

Street drugs   *Psychoactive drugs* manufactured and sold illegally.

Stupor   A state of reduced sensibility, often the result of excessive use of *depressants*.

Subcutaneous   Under the skin, such as the injection of a drug just under the skin rather than into a muscle or vein.

Subtoxic   Below the toxic dose of a drug.

Super-K   Slang term for ketamine.

Sympathetic nervous system   That branch of the involuntary nervous system that prepares the body for fight or flight by speeding up heart-beat and breathing, and at the same time shutting down digestive functions. Nerves of this system leave the middle segments of the spinal cord to connect to many organs, blood vessels, and glands.

Synergism   In pharmacology, the interaction of two drugs to produce a combined effect greater than the simple sum of their individual effects.

Synthetic drugs   Drugs created by chemists in laboratories, as opposed to *endogenous drugs* or *semisynthetic drugs*.

Taboo   A prohibition excluding something from use or mention, devised by any group for its own protection.

Teetotaler   A person who abstains totally from drinking alcohol.

Testosterone   The principal male sex hormone, manufactured by the testes and responsible for producing male sex characteristics.

Therapeutic   Having healing or curative powers.

Tincture   A solution of a substance, especially a drug, in alcohol.

Toke   An inhalation from a cigarette or pipe. Also used as a verb.

Tolerance   In pharmacology, the need for increasing doses of a drug over time to maintain the same effect. Tolerance is an important characteristic of dependence on drugs and is provoked by some drugs more than others, especially by *stimulants* and *depressants*.

Toxic   Poisonous. Harmful, destructive, or deadly.

Trafficking   In drug law, the distribution, sale, exchange, or giving away of significant amounts of prohibited substances; considered a more serious crime than simple possession.

Trip   An experience on a *psychoactive drug*, especially a *hallucinogen*.

Underground chemist   A chemist who manufactures *psychoactive drugs* illegally for sale on the black market.

Uppers   *Stimulants.*

Users   1) People who use *psychoactive drugs*. 2) People who use psychoactive drugs in nonabusive ways, as opposed to *abusers*.

Visions   Mental images produced in the imagination, usually seen with the eyes closed; also, the mystical experience of seeing other realities or the supernatural as if with the eyes.

Volatile   Evaporating rapidly at normal temperatures and pressures.

Windowpane   Slang term for LSD in the form of tiny, transparent gelatin chips.

Withdrawal   1) The process of stopping the use of a drug that has been taken regularly. 2) Any cluster of symptoms that appears when a drug that has been taken regularly is stopped and that disappears when the drug is reinstituted. Also called a withdrawal syndrome.

Index